Professionalism in Health Care

A Primer for Career Success

4TH EDITION

Sherry Makely, PhD, R.T.(R)
Pine Ridge Publications
Bloomington, Indiana

Contributing Authors

Vanessa J. Austin, RMA, AHI, (AMT), MS
Sanford Brown College
Indianapolis, Indiana

Quay Kester, PhD
Evoke Communications
Indianapolis, Indiana

PEARSON

Boston Columbus Indianapolis New York San Francisco Upper Saddle River
Amsterdam Cape Town Dubai London Madrid Milan Munich Paris Montréal Toronto
Delhi Mexico City São Paulo Sydney Hong Kong Seoul Singapore Taipei Tokyo

Publisher: Julie Levin Alexander
Publisher's Assistant: Regina Bruno
Editor-in-Chief: Mark Cohen
Executive Editor: Joan Gill
Associate Editor: Melissa Kerian
Editorial Assistant: Mary Ellen Ruitenberg
Director of Marketing: David Gesell
Marketing Manager: Katrin Beacom
Marketing Specialist: Michael Sirinides
Marketing Assistant: Crystal Gonzalez
Managing Production Editor: Patrick Walsh

Production Liaison: Julie Boddorf
Senior Media Editor: Amy Peltier
Media Project Manager: Lorena Cerisano
Manufacturing Manager: Lisa McDowell
Senior Art Director: Maria Guglielmo
Interior Design: Element Thomson North America
Cover Designer: Wanda España, Wee Design
Cover Photo: ©wavebreakmedia ltd/Shutterstock
Composition: Element Thomson North America
Printing and Binding: Quad/Graphics-Taunton
Cover Printer: Lehigh-Phoenix Color

Library of Congress Cataloging-in-Publication Data
Makely, Sherry.
   Professionalism in health care : a primer for career success / Sherry Makely, Vanessa J. Austin, Quay Kester. — 4th ed.
      p. ; cm.
   Includes index.
   ISBN 978-0-13-284010-1
   I. Austin, Vanessa   J. II. Kester, Quay.   III. Title.
   [DNLM: 1. Health Occupations.   2. Professional Competence.   3. Career Mobility.
4. Ethics, Professional.   5. Interprofessional Relations. W 21]
   LC-classification not assigned
   610.69—dc23

2011031152

10 9 8 7 6 5 4 3 2 1

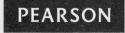

ISBN 10: 0-13-284010-3
ISBN 13: 978-0-13284010-1

Contents

Preface   vi

Reviewers   x

About the Authors   xi

Acknowledgments   xii

Health Care Professionals   xiii

Introduction   xiv

Chapter One The Health Care Industry and Your Role   1

Working in Health Care   2

Health Care as a Business   7

Impact of the Baby Boomer Population   9

Improving the Nation's Health Care System   10

The Big Picture and Where You Fit In   20

Learning Activities   22

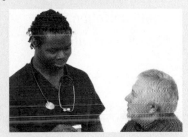

Chapter Two Your Work Ethic and Performance   27

Making a Commitment to Your Job   28

Developing a Strong Work Ethic   32

Representing Your Employer   41

Evaluating Your Performance   43

Learning Activities   48

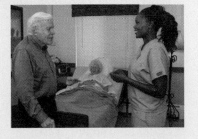

**Chapter Three Personal Traits of the Health Care
            Professional   53**

Character and Personal Values   54

Character Traits   55

Reputation   58

Judgment   58

Conscience   59

Trust   60

Honesty   61

Ethics   64

Ethical, Moral, and Legal Dilemmas   66

Learning Activities   68

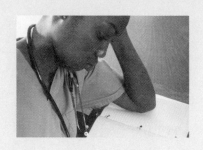

Chapter Four Relationships, Teamwork, and Communication Skills   73

Interpersonal Relationships   74

Teams and Teamwork   81

Communication Skills   84

Learning Activities   95

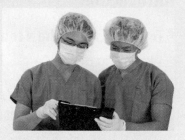

Chapter Five Cultural Competence and Patient Care   100

Quay Kester, PhD

Diversity and Culture   101

Working with Patients   110

Working with Doctors, Guests,
   and Vendors   119

Learning Activities   122

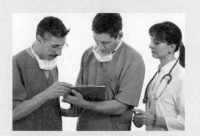

Chapter Six Professionalism and Your Personal Life   127

Personal Image   128

Personal Health and Wellness   137

Personal Management Skills   139

Learning Activities   144

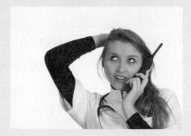

Chapter Seven The Practicum Experience   150

Vanessa J. Austin

The Purpose of a Practicum   151

The Benefits of a Practicum Experience   151

Preparing for Your Practicum   154

During Your Practicum   156

Ensuring Success on Your Practicum   164

After Your Practicum   165

Learning Activities   167

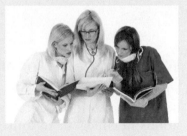

Chapter Eight Employment, Leadership, and Career Development   172

Job-Seeking Skills   173

Applying for Jobs   180

Interviews   185

Becoming a Professional Leader   193

Career Development   197

Learning Activities   204

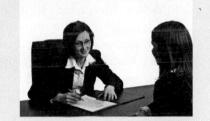

In Summary   209

Glossary of Terms   210

Appendices

A: Sample Job Description   219

B: Sample Performance Evaluation   221

C: Sample Résumé   224

D: Sample Résumé Cover Letter   226

E: Sample Job Application Form   227

F: Sample Interview Follow-Up Letter   231

G: Sample Practicum Journal   232

H: Sample Practicum Thank You Letter   234

Index   235

Preface

Who This Book Is for and Why It's Important

Professionalism in Health Care: A Primer for Career Success, 4th Edition, is designed for students enrolled in nursing and health sciences educational programs in colleges and universities, vocational-technical schools, hospitals, high schools, and on-the-job training programs. This book is also beneficial in orientation sessions for new employees and for in-service and refresher classes for experienced health care workers. Text information is applicable to all health careers and all types, sizes, and locations of health care settings including hospitals, clinics, outpatient facilities, occupational health centers, dental practices, rehabilitation centers, physician practices, surgery centers, home care agencies, mental health facilities, pharmacies, community health centers, nursing homes, transitional and long-term care facilities, satellite imaging and laboratory facilities, public health organizations, urgent care centers, and insurance and billing companies.

This book provides information that is essential to the success of today's health care workers. Hands-on technical skills remain a high priority but good character, a strong work ethic, and personal and professional traits and behaviors are becoming more important than ever before. Statistics indicate a growing concern with theft, fraud, and behavioral problems in the workplace. Poor attendance, interpersonal conflicts, disregard for quality, and disrespect for authority all too often lead to employees being fired from their jobs. With a growing emphasis on customer service, patient satisfaction, cultural competence, quality improvement, patient safety, and corporate compliance, health care employers are increasingly seeking workers with strong "soft skills" and "people skills"—people who communicate appropriately, work well on teams, respect and value differences, use limited resources efficiently, and interact effectively with coworkers, patients, and guests.

Regardless of job title or discipline, every health care student and worker must understand the importance of professionalism and the need to perform in a professional, ethical, legal, and competent manner. Developing and strengthening professional traits and behaviors has become a major challenge for both health care educators and employers. This book helps meet that challenge. It describes professional standards that apply to all health care workers—the common ground that everyone shares in providing the highest quality of health care and service excellence for patients, visitors, and guests.

What This Book Covers

Professionalism in Health Care: A Primer for Career Success, 4th Edition, discusses the following:

- Key elements of professionalism
- The health care industry and your role
- Your work ethic and performance
- Personal and character traits
- Relationships, teamwork, and communication skills
- Cultural competence and patient care
- Professionalism and your personal life
- The practicum experience
- Employment, leadership, and career development

New to This Edition

This fourth edition includes a new full-color layout; updated, new, and expanded content; and several new features:

- A new Chapter One, "The Health Care Industry and Your Role," discusses current trends and issues in health care with implications for health care workers. Topics include working in health care, health care as a business, impact of the baby boomer population, improving the nation's health care system, health care reform efforts, electronic medical records, and the "big picture" and where health care workers fit in. Over 60 glossary terms are presented in this new chapter.
- Chapter Three in the third edition, "Working with Others" has been split into two chapters in the fourth edition, "Relationships, Teamwork, and Communication Skills" and "Cultural Competence and Patient Care" to enhance the content.
- Topics and content have been expanded throughout the 4th edition chapters. Expanded topics include critical thinking and problem-solving skills, quality improvement, patient safety, character traits, cultural competence, customer service, manners and etiquette, electronic communication, employment and interviewing skills, leadership skills, career development, and technologic innovations to improve patient care.
- Each chapter has several new features: Think About It, Recent Developments, and Consider This present current trends and issues related to chapter content. Key Points summarize chapter content and Reality Check brings the message home to the reader. For More Information provides additional resources. The case study illustrates how chapter content applies to a fictional medical assistant's career.
- Two new appendixes have been added, "Sample Practicum Journal" and "Sample Practicum Thank-You Letter."

- One hundred and forty-eight new glossary terms and definitions have been added for a total of 263 terms.

Another new feature of this fourth edition is the companion website. Content and resources from the Student CD-ROM, Instructor CD-ROM, and *Instructor Resource Manual* included with the third edition of the textbook are now available on the new website located at www.myhealthprofessionskit.com.

The student portion of the website presents additional learning opportunities that include several videos with scenarios that are applicable to all types of health care workers in a variety of employment and patient care settings. New in the fourth edition is the Golden Personality Type Profiler presented in the website content for Chapter Five. This workplace personality assessment provides information to help explain why an individual behaves in a certain way in workplace situations and how people respond to stress at work.

The instructor portion of the new website includes the *Instructor Resource Manual* and electronic content that can be used in classroom courses or downloaded onto an online learning environment for instructor-facilitated courses as well as independent study courses.

The *Instructor Resource Manual* includes the following:

- Guidelines for using the material for classroom, online, and self-study courses
- Suggestions for using PowerPoint slides, sample documents, and other resources
- Course description, course objectives, and chapter objectives
- A large test bank with answers mapped to text material
- Chapter lesson plans with discussion topics and recommended learning experiences
- Answers to Chapter Review Questions and What If? Scenarios in the text
- Answers to website questions and quizzes

The *Instructor's Resource Manual* also provides an independent study guide to assist in developing online and independent study courses. Used in conjunction with the textbook and website, the independent study guide provides a self-paced or structured approach as determined by the facilitator.

Information for Students

Students should read each chapter in the textbook and complete the end-of-chapter learning activities prior to moving on to the next chapter. End-of-chapter learning activities include Chapter Review Questions and What If? Scenarios. Based on course requirements, students may also complete website activities including Scenario Analysis Quizzes, Self-Assessments, Next Step Improvement Plans, Learning Opportunities, and other chapter-specific activities.

Information for Instructors

This textbook is designed for use in (1) classroom-based, instructor-led courses, (2) instructor-facilitated online courses, and (3) independent study courses. The book may also be used for (1) personal reading for self-instruction and review, (2) orientation and training for new health care workers, and (3) in-service and continuing education seminars for experienced health care workers. The textbook and website materials may be incorporated into introductory, core curriculum, and capstone courses in nursing and the health sciences. The material may also be used as practicum preparation and for workshops on topics such as employment strategies, career development, and work readiness. Instructors may choose to use this text in a general introductory course and then supplement learning through an advanced, discipline-specific course later on.

In Closing

We hope you find *Professionalism in Health Care: A Primer for Career Success, 4th Edition,* and its companion website informative, thought provoking, and beneficial.

Reviewers

Tamra J. Ashley
RN, MSN, CFNP, IBCLC
Departmental Coordinator
Davenport University
Lansing, Michigan

Karen Betts, MA
Associate Academic Dean
Concorde Career College
San Diego, California

Michelle Buchman, MA, BSN, RN
Medical Assisting Program
Coordinator and Assistant Professor
Cox College
Springfield, Missouri

Michele M. Buzard,
MS, MT(ASCP), BA
Phlebotomy Program Director
Kaplan University-Hagerstown
Hagerstown, Maryland

Paula L. Griswold, PhD,
MT(ASCP), CPC(AAPC)
Assistant Professor and
Practicum Coordinator
University of Louisiana at Monroe
Monroe, Louisiana

Brigitte Niedzwiecki RN, MSN
Medical Assistant Program
Director and Instructor
Chippewa Valley Technical College
Eau Claire, Wisconsin

Julie Pepper, CMA(AAMA)
Instructor, Medical Assisting
Chippewa Valley Technical College
Eau Claire, Wisconsin

Teresa Rivers
Part-time Adjunct Instructor
Warren County Career Center
Lebanon, Ohio

About The Authors

Sherry Makely, PhD, R.T.(R) Textbook Author

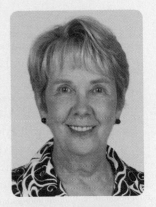

Dr. Makely has created and managed health sciences educational programs and workforce development initiatives in hospitals and universities for over 42 years. She has a bachelor's degree in radiologic technology, a master's degree in education, and a doctorate degree in human resources. Dr. Makely served as director of education of the School of Radiologic Science and manager of the Employee Education and Development Department for Methodist Hospital, Clarian Health, and Indiana University Health for 38 years prior to joining the Health Care Pathways Development Team at Pearson Workforce Education in 2011.

Vanessa J. Austin, RMA, AHI, (AMT), MS Contributing Author, "The Practicum Experience," Chapter Seven

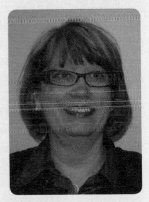

With more than 15 years experience as a medical assistant and clinical education coordinator of Clarian Health's Medical Assisting Program in Indianapolis, Indiana, Ms. Austin serves as medical assisting clinical coordinator at Sanford Brown College Indianapolis. With a bachelor's degree in health care management and a master's degree in higher education, she speaks on the topic of professionalism in health care for state and national conferences and serves as president of the Indiana State Society of American Medical Technologists.

Quay Kester, PhD Content Contributor, "Cultural Competence," Chapter Five

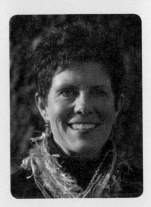

Dr. Quay Kester, president of Evoke Communications, specializes in diversity and inclusion initiatives to build cultural competence and confidence in health care, academic, and corporate organizations. Her avid commitment to learning about cultures and customs has taken her throughout the world working with various populations in developing countries. Her national and international experience makes her a sought-after speaker, leader, and facilitator. Dr. Kester has served as adjunct faculty at Indiana University, DePauw University, and as visiting professor at the University of Cape Coast, Ghana. With a doctorate degree from Indiana University, she is a master practitioner of neurolinguistic programming and a certified medical illustrator. She serves as an educator and consultant for Indiana University Health and as a member of numerous boards including the Diversity Roundtable of Central Indiana.

Acknowledgments

Appreciation is extended to photographer Carmen Martin and the following individuals who appear in textbook and website photographs:

Tracey Alcorn
Xochitl Alejandre
Shakira Alexander
Vanessa Austin
Kelley Beagle
Jodi Blevins
Ashlee Boggs
J'Anthanee Bonner
Terry Brooks-Allen
Kathy Chlystun
Cecilia Curtin
Iesha Dinwiddie
Christopher Gerth
Meaza Ghebresilassie
Melissa Gilliland
Rustyna Hodo
Edward Hollins
Raelyna Huddleston
Damon Hynds
Madonna Key

Debbie Landrey
Michael Levine
Carmen Martin
Estela Martinez
Cheri McKinney
Kimberly Milstead
Andrew Mong
Jennifer Olson
Rosaura Sanchez
Shanica Short
Dinh Sizemore
Corey Smith
Joan Stewart
Jeremy Tarter
Soulena Teague
Sara Unthank
Terri Vandermark
Shannon Washington
Don Weir
Marsha Wilson

Health Care Professionals

Recognition as a health care professional is something that has to be earned—a reputation that's developed and maintained each and every day you come to work. Professionalism is a state of mind, a way of "being," "knowing," and "doing" that sets you apart from others. It gives direction to how you look, behave, think, and act. It brings together who you are as a person, what you value, how you treat other people, what you contribute in the workplace, and how seriously you take your job. Professionals don't just work to earn a paycheck. Income is important but professionals view their work as a source of pride and a reflection of the role they play in society.

Health care professionals are good at what they do—and they like doing it. They enjoy helping others and knowing they've made a difference. Professionals have their "act together"—and it shows. They set high standards for their performance and achieve them. They see the "big picture" in health care and know where they fit in. Professionals care about quality and how to improve it. They treat everyone they meet with dignity and respect. And they continually strive to grow and to learn.

Introduction

Opportunity is missed by most because it is dressed in overalls and looks like work.

Thomas Alva Edison, Inventor, 1847–1931

KEY TERMS

accreditation	diagnostic	practicum	scope of practice
attitude	dignity	professional associations	self-esteem
caregivers	hierarchy	professionals	self-worth
certifications	licenses	providers	therapeutic
competence	outpatient	reputation	trust
credentials	payers	respect	vendors

Recognition as a Health Care Professional

There's no doubt about it. When you're sick or injured or when a family member or friend needs health care you want to be certain that you and your loved ones are cared for by **professionals** (people with experience and skills who are engaged in a specific occupation for pay or as a means of livelihood). Thinking back to the times when you've had a doctor's appointment, visited an outpatient clinic (a place to receive medical care without being admitted to a hospital) or emergency department, or have been hospitalized for tests or treatments, you probably encountered many different types of health care workers. Although most of these workers performed their duties in a professional manner, you may have encountered a few who did not. We would like to think that everyone who works in health care functions as a professional but experience has shown that such is not always the case.

What is a professional? How can you recognize a professional when you see one? What does "taking a professional approach" to one's work mean? Why is professionalism important? What must you learn as a student to prepare for future recognition as a health care professional yourself?

According to *Webster's New World Dictionary of the American Language, College Edition*, a *professional* is a person "with much experience and great skill in a specified role" who is "engaged in a specific occupation for pay or as a means of livelihood." As we look around us, we see many examples of professionals in different walks of life. In sports, for example, professional status is awarded to gifted athletes who have surpassed amateur events and moved into high-paying, major league competitions. In medicine, law, and science, doctors, lawyers, and engineers are considered professionals because of their expertise, college education, and special **credentials** (a letter or certificate given to a person to show that he or she has the right to exercise a certain authority) such as **licenses** (credentials from a state agency awarding legal permission to practice; must meet pre-established qualifications) and **certifications** (credentials from a state agency or a professional association awarding permission to use a special professional title; must meet pre-established competency standards). But truck drivers, hair stylists, and photographers consider themselves as professionals, too, as do bankers, insurance underwriters, and investment counselors. Exactly what is a professional and who is qualified to be one?

Occupations are sometimes divided into professional and nonprofessional categories based on criteria such as the following:

- Unique and exclusive **scope of practice** (boundaries that determine what a worker may and may not do as part of his or her job)
- Minimum educational standards and **accreditation** (certified as having met set standards) of educational programs
- Minimum standards for entry into practice
- Required credentials such as licenses or certifications
- **Professional associations** (organizations composed of people from the same occupation) with codes of ethics and standards of **competence** (possessing necessary knowledge and skills)

When we apply these criteria to the health care workforce, then doctors, registered nurses, pharmacists, physical therapists, medical assistants, surgical technologists, dental assistants, radiographers, and the like are all classified as professionals. But that leaves other types of health care workers such as insurance processors, food service workers, housekeepers, and equipment repair technicians in the nonprofessional classification. Not making the list of professionals can be demeaning to people who work hard and make their jobs a top priority in their lives.

In health care it's important to acknowledge another set of criteria that gives all health care workers the opportunity to be viewed as professionals whether they provide direct patient care or function in a support role behind the scenes: it's not *the job you do* that makes you a professional, it's *how you do your job* that counts.

Every health care worker has the opportunity—and the obligation—to strive for professional recognition. Regardless of how other people may classify your job as professional or nonprofessional, always remember that it's what you contribute in the workplace that really matters.

Professional recognition isn't something that's automatically bestowed on a person when he or she completes an educational program, obtains a degree or certificate, or secures a license to practice. It's not dependent on a person's socioeconomic status, income, age, gender, race, job title, or position within the **hierarchy** (a group of people or units arranged by rank) of an organization. After all, we've all known people with college degrees, special credentials, and impressive job titles who don't behave in a professional manner.

Recognition as a health care professional is something that has to be earned—a **reputation** (a person's character, values, and behavior as viewed by others) that's developed and maintained each and every day you come to work. Professionalism is a state of mind, a way of "being," "knowing," and "doing" that sets you apart from others. It gives direction to how you look, behave, think, and act. It brings together who you are as a person, what you value, how you treat other people, what you contribute in the workplace, and how seriously you take your job. Professionals don't just work to earn a paycheck. Income is important but professionals view their work as a source of pride and a reflection of the role they play in society.

If you're serious about a career in health care, viewing yourself as a professional and being recognized as such by other people will be a major key to your success. Professionalism is something every organization looks for in its employees. How can you spot a health care professional when you see one? It's easy.

Health care professionals are good at what they do—and they like doing it. They enjoy helping others and knowing they've made a difference. Professionals "have their act together"—and it shows. They set high standards for their performance and achieve them. They see the "big picture" in health care and know where they fit in. Professionals care about quality and how to improve it. They treat everyone they meet with **dignity** (the degree of worth, merit, honor) and **respect** (feeling or showing honor or esteem). They continually strive to grow and to learn.

Spotting a health care professional may be easy but becoming one yourself is another matter. It's something you have to concentrate on every day but it's worth it. To *be* a professional, you must *feel like* a professional. In our society, the amount of education a person has and what he or she does for a living have become important contributors to an individual's **self-esteem** (belief in oneself, self-respect) and sense of **self-worth** (importance and value in oneself). *What we do* has become *who we are*. When you graduate from an educational program, earn a degree, or obtain a license or certification you experience the exhilaration of knowing you've accomplished something worthwhile. Being recognized by others as a professional brings value and meaning to your efforts. It reminds you that what you do really counts. This is true whether you care for patients, process specimens, prepare meals, clean public areas, interact with **vendors** (people who work for companies with which your company does business) or work in any one of hundreds of different health care jobs. It's also true whether you work in a hospital, physicians' office, dental

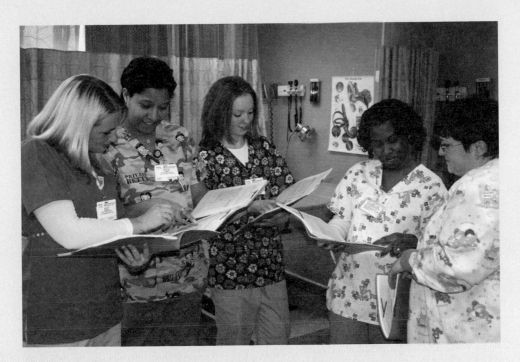

practice, clinic, rehab facility, or some other type of health care organization. No matter what your role involves, how you view your work and how you approach it can have a tremendous impact on your own life as well as on the lives of those you serve.

Why Health Care Needs Professionals

When you are sick or injured, health care can become a basic need for survival. Each year, millions of Americans receive health services in doctors' offices, hospitals, clinics, mental health facilities, and in their homes. Patients rely on health care professionals to provide affordable, state-of-the-art **diagnostic** (deciding the nature of a disease or condition) and **therapeutic** (treating or curing a disease or condition) procedures to help them overcome illness, injury, and other abnormalities that affect their health and quality of life.

It's important to keep in mind that health care is a business. Finding ways to provide health care for more patients, using fewer resources, while achieving better outcomes has become a major challenge for health care **providers** (doctors, health care workers, and health care organizations that offer health care services) and **payers** (someone that covers the expense for goods received or services rendered). Meeting these challenges requires a cadre of health care workers who are committed to quality care, customer service, and cost effectiveness. People who fail to take a professional approach to their work are often late, absent, unreliable, and sloppy. Their actions may endanger patient care, customer service, safety, and the efficient use of limited resources.

Working in health care requires special skills and an **attitude** (a manner of acting, feeling, or thinking that shows one's disposition or opinion) that supports service to others. Patients seek health care services during some of the most vulnerable times in their lives, when they're sick, injured, and "at their worst." Each patient-worker interaction must build confidence and **trust** (to place confidence in the honesty, integrity, and reliability of another person). The decisions and actions of those who care for patients or those who work behind the scenes to support the efforts of **caregivers** (health care workers who provide direct, hands-on patient care) can have an immediate and lasting impact.

The Importance of Every Job and Every Worker

Regardless of what type of job you are preparing for, you will play an important role in health care because every job and every worker is important. Let's face reality—if a job weren't important it wouldn't exist.

It should be obvious that professionalism is vital in every job. Your challenge is to pull together the mixture of knowledge, skills, compassion, and commitment required to make you the very best employee you can possibly be. If you can meet this challenge every day on the job, then you've earned the privilege of being recognized as a health care professional. Nothing less is acceptable.

The information in this text will help guide your journey to professional recognition. It's important to start developing your reputation now while you are still a student. Apply yourself, take your studies seriously, learn to manage your time, and hone your communication skills. Make thoughtful decisions, encourage and support your fellow classmates, and find ways to balance the priorities in your life. Remember that everything that you hear, observe, learn, and experience will be important at some point in your health career. If your educational program includes a **practicum** (a "real-life" learning experience obtained through working on-site in a health care facility while enrolled as a student; also known as clinicals, externship, internship, hands-on experience, and so on), you'll be interacting with health care workers, physicians, and patients to gain hands-on experience even before you graduate.

Expect some changes along the way, plan to continue your learning after you graduate from school, and always strive to do your very best. You and the patients you will some day serve deserve nothing less.

The Health Care Industry and Your Role

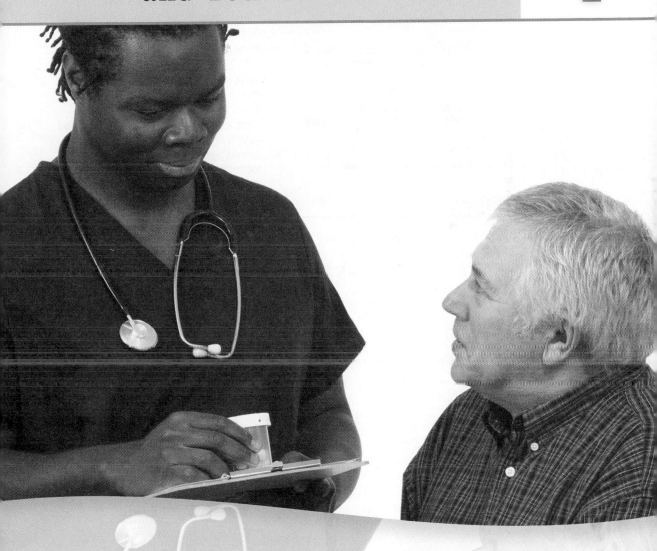

"In a world that is constantly changing, there is no one subject or set of subjects that will serve you for the foreseeable future, let alone for the rest of your life. The most important skill to acquire now is learning how to learn."

John Naisbitt,
International best-selling author, 1929–present

CHAPTER OBJECTIVES

Having completed this chapter, you will be able to:

- List four benefits of working in the health care industry.
- Define *soft skills* and *hard skills*, explain the difference, and discuss why both are important.
- List two reasons why it's important for health care professionals to know about current trends and issues in the health care industry.
- List three reasons why health care is expensive and the cost continues to rise.

- Identify four ways that the baby boomer population will impact the health care industry.
- Identify and discuss two controversial issues associated with health care reform.
- Define *continuous quality improvement* and list two quality improvement goals.
- Define *sentinel event* and explain the connection between sentinel events and patient safety.
- Identify two trends in the supply and demand of health care workers.
- List two advantages and disadvantages of electronic medical records.

KEY TERMS

accountability	defensive medicine	interpersonal skills	preexisting condition
accountable care organizations (ACOs)	discipline	legibility	prenatal
	diverse	life expectancy	preventive
acute	donut hole	malpractice	primary care
adverse effects	emotional intelligence quotient (EQ)	managed care	process
alternative medicine		Medicaid	readmission
baby boomers	empowered	medical homes	root cause
baseline data	EMRs	Medicare	sentinel event
breach	error	metrics	single-payer system
capitation	gatekeepers	mistake	Six Sigma
chronic	geriatric	multiskilled	soft skills
complementary medicine	gross domestic product (GDP)	obese	specialists
		outcome data	staffing level
confidentiality	hard skills	out-of-pocket expense	stakeholders
consumers	health care exchanges		traits
continuity	individual mandate	people skills	transferable skills
continuous quality improvement (CQI)	infant mortality rate	personality	universal health care
	intelligence quotient (IQ)	perspective	work ethic

Working in Health Care

Whether you are preparing for your first job or gaining the knowledge and skills you need for career advancement, you've made a good decision choosing a health care occupation. Working in health care offers many benefits and opportunities.

Job opportunities now and in the future appear excellent. Although the 2008 recession eliminated millions of jobs throughout the United States, jobs in the health care sector grew steadily. Since late 2007, the number of non-health care jobs dropped by almost 7% while the number of health care jobs increased by 6.3%. Most of the new health care jobs were in outpatient settings such as doctors' offices and clinics. Even during the post-recession recovery that started in June 2009, non-health care employment continued to decline as heath care employment increased every month.

Health care employs about 10% of all U.S. workers. Ten of the 20 fastest-growing occupations are in health care, and this trend is likely to continue because of the rapid growth of the elderly population. In fact, between now and the year 2018, health care will generate more new jobs than any other industry.

The health care industry offers **diverse** (different, varied) employment opportunities, ranging from small town physician practices with one medical assistant to large, urban academic medical centers and health systems employing thousands of workers. Many employers offer flexible work schedules and most provide valuable benefits such as health and life insurance, paid vacation time and holidays, tuition assistance, and a retirement plan.

With so many different occupations from which to choose, health care workers have an abundance of opportunities for career advancement. You can:

- Earn advanced degrees and additional professional certifications
- Move up the ladder in your original **discipline** (a branch of knowledge or learning such as nursing, medical assisting, surgical technology, etc.)
- Become **multiskilled** (cross-trained to perform more than one function, often in more than one discipline)
- Apply your **transferable skills** (skills acquired in one job that are applicable in another job) to train in a different discipline
- Advance into leadership, teaching, sales, or research jobs

One of best benefits of working in health care is the opportunity to improve the quality of people's lives. As mentioned in the Introduction, when you are sick or injured health care can become a basic need for survival. People seek health care services during some of the most vulnerable times in their lives. Premature babies struggle to survive, injured athletes strive to regain strength, people with **acute** (severe but over a short period of time) and **chronic** (occurs frequently over a long period of time) ailments try to lead normal lives, and terminally ill patients face end-of-life decisions. Health care workers are at their patients' sides from cradle to grave, providing crucial diagnostic and therapeutic procedures, compassionate care, and helpful encouragement and support. It's a privilege to work in health care and touch the lives of everyone you serve.

As a service industry, health care requires superb **people skills** (personality characteristics that enhance your ability to interact effectively with other

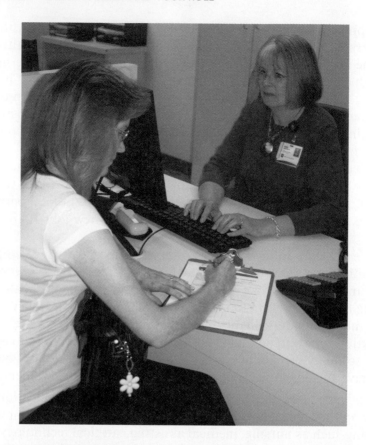

Figure 1-1 ■ Patient checking in at registration

people) as well as technical competence. Employers call these **soft skills**—the **personality** characteristics that enhance your ability to interact effectively with other people. Soft skills and **interpersonal skills** (the ability to interact with other people) enhance your relationships, job performance, and career prospects. Sometimes referred to as your **emotional intelligence quotient** or **EQ** (the ability to perceive, assess, and manage your own emotions and other people's emotions), soft skills relate more to *who you are* than *what you know*—your **intelligence quotient** or **IQ** (the ability to learn, understand, and deal with new and trying situations). Once you've graduated from your educational program and have obtained credentials to practice, employers will assume you are competent to perform the hands-on, technical, **hard skills** duties of your job. Hard skills can be learned and improved over time but soft skills are part of your personality and are much more difficult to acquire and change. Employers are increasingly screening, hiring, paying, and promoting for soft skills to ensure that their employees work harmoniously with other people.

This book focuses on the soft skills you need to achieve success in health care. The book discusses the following:

- **Work ethic** (attitudes and behaviors that support good work performance)
- Personal and character **traits** (characteristics or qualities related to one's personality)
- Relationships and communication skills
- Working with patients and customer service
- Professionalism and your personal life
- The practicum experience
- Employment and career advancement

Before addressing these topics, let's focus on another important step in preparing for a role in health care—learning as much as you can about the industry's current trends and issues. As a health care worker, you'll be part of the nation's fastest growing industry. You'll need to consider questions such as these:

- How much do you know about the health care industry?
- Are you up to speed with current topics and know where health care is headed?
- Do you know enough about local and national health care issues to discuss them intelligently with other people?

Everyone is affected by the health care industry, and many Americans have opinions about what's wrong with health care and how to fix it. This is especially true today because health care has become very expensive. All Americans, and especially health care workers, need to be actively involved in finding ways to make improvements.

If you want to be viewed as a health care professional, you need to be aware of what's going on in your industry. This doesn't mean you have to be a walking encyclopedia on health care terminology and all of the topics under debate, but you do need to keep up with current trends and issues and consider how they might affect your job, your patients, your personal health, and your career. Be on the lookout for information from a variety of sources. Read articles about health care in magazines, newspapers, medical journals, and online sources. Watch the news on television and look for special programs about health care. Attend health care seminars and conferences when you get the opportunity and become active in your discipline's professional organizations. Speak with people who are current on the latest trends and join in conversations to discuss the issues.

By deciding to work in health care, you have chosen an industry like no other. Consider the following:

- Workers are dealing with life-and-death situations on a daily basis, 24/7/365.
- Things are changing rapidly; new devices, drugs, and medical procedures are under development every day.

CASE STUDY

Carla graduated from her medical assisting program just over a year ago. After considering three job offers, she decided to work in a small practice owned by three family medicine doctors. One of the doctors is nearing retirement age, another has 10 years of experience, and the third just completed his medical residency program about two years ago.

Things were going just fine until last week when the practice manager and doctors announced that changes on are the way. They said they need to find ways to care for more patients, especially those covered by Medicare. They want to prepare for the impact of health care reform, adjust to changes in health insurance, replace outdated equipment, remodel the waiting area and exam rooms, employ a physician assistant and another nurse practitioner, and have more control over their income and expenses to remain competitive and financially sound. They said that, after a great deal of thought, they've decided to give up their private practice and join a network.

Within six months, the name of the practice will change and the employees, including Carla, will be working for the network company. Patient medical records, currently stored in paper files, will be transferred to **EMRs** (electronic medical records.) Doctors and staff will undergo training to use sophisticated computer software to store medical histories, physical exam information, and treatment notes; order blood tests, x-rays, and other procedures; locate and evaluate test results; send prescriptions to the pharmacy; and provide immediate access to complete, up-to-date medical information when their patients receive services in other locations.

What do these changes mean for Carla? She chose this practice because of its small size and relatively low-stress environment. She has basic computer skills but is worried about having to master new technology. She can't help but wonder if these changes are really necessary. Carla's former classmate, who works at another nearby medical practice, said they have an opening for a medical assistant (MA) and nothing has been said in her practice about joining a network or switching to EMRs.

Should Carla stay or look for another job? If she decides to stay, what could she do to prepare for the changes? Could she help her doctors, manager, and coworkers make the transition? What might happen if she leaves? What would you do if you were Carla?

- Hospitals and doctors are forming networks, restructuring organizations, and redesigning jobs and job duties.
- Population trends, especially the aging of **baby boomers** (people born in the United States between 1946 and 1964), are driving major changes in health care.
- An insufficient supply of doctors and health care workers in rural areas and economically depressed urban areas are leaving large segments of the population medically underserved.

When you consider all of these factors, it becomes clear that change is the name of the game in health care. It's a fast-moving train. You need to climb onboard or risk being left behind. You must know what's going on and where things appear to be headed so you can be well informed and prepared for the future.

Health care has become one of the most controversial industries in recent years, with multiple issues and concerns under debate. Can the United States retool its health care system so that everyone who needs health care can access medical services at an affordable cost? Health care is a business. As a health care professional, it's important to know about the business side of your industry and where you fit in.

Health Care as a Business

Most of what you'll learn in this book relates to working in a patient care environment—the service side of the health care industry—but understanding the business side of health care is important, too. Health care is expensive, it's a necessity of life, and it affects everyone including **consumers** (people who purchase or use a product or service), taxpayers, employers, businesses, government, and other **stakeholders** (people with a keen interest in a project or organization; may be end-users of a product or service). Consider the following:

- As patients, everyone is a consumer of health care. When the need arises, consumers want the best health care available regardless of the cost.
- As taxpayers, everyone pays for health care through programs such as **Medicare** (a government program that provides health care primarily for people 65 and older) and **Medicaid** (a government program that provides health care for low-income people and families and for people with certain disabilities).
- The United States spends about $2.5 trillion per year (about $8,500 per person) on health care, significantly more than any other developed nation, and the cost is rising about 8% a year.
- Unpaid medical bills are a leading cause of bankruptcy in the United States.
- Health care costs account for about 18% of the nation's **gross domestic product (GDP)** and are rising (GDP is the total market value of all good and services produced in one year).

So when it comes to health care, everyone is a stakeholder with concerns and opinions to voice.

Providing health care for everyone who needs it at a reasonable expense is an enormous challenge. The cost of health care in the United States is growing faster than the cost of most other goods and services. Cost increases result from:

- The need to recruit, pay, and retain highly competent doctors and health professionals

- Medical research to develop new drugs, devices, and medical procedures
- Rising cost of medical equipment, supplies, and utilities
- Building construction, remodeling, and maintenance
- The expense of training future doctors, nurses, and other health professionals

As the cost of health care increases, Americans are voicing their concerns about health insurance and how to pay for it. People who have health insurance usually receive coverage through their employer, a government program such as Medicare or Medicaid, or an individual or group policy. Each patient has a **primary care** doctor who provides the basic medical care that a person receives upon first contact with the health care system. The primary care doctor then refers the patient to a variety of **specialists** depending on the additional services needed. With primary care doctors acting as **gatekeepers** (people who monitor the actions of other people and who control access to something), the goal is to:

- Encourage **preventive** services (actions taken to avoid a medical condition) such as vaccinations, flu shots, and health screenings
- Provide medical care in the least expensive settings such as doctors' offices, outpatient clinics, and the patient's home
- Avoid unnecessary or duplicate tests and treatments
- Coordinate services from different providers to ensure **continuity** (continuous, uninterrupted, and connected) in care and the best outcomes for the patient

Controlling the cost of health care is just one of the problems. Ensuring adequate access to health care services is also a concern. Millions of Americans don't have health insurance or a primary care doctor. They go without medical care or rely on hospital emergency departments where the cost of caring for patients is very high. They go without prescription drugs, which makes their conditions more difficult and expensive to treat in the long run. Pregnant women forego **prenatal** care (occurring before birth) which can cause major problems later on.

When patients are unable (or unwilling) to pay their medical bills, the providers must write off the loss as charity care or unreimbursed services. Since hospitals and doctors have to cover their expenses to remain in business, this loss of income drives up the cost for other patients who do have health insurance and who do pay their bills.

The lack of doctors and medical facilities in rural areas and in medically underserved urban areas also limits access to health care services for many Americans. Many doctors and health care professionals prefer to live and work in attractive urban areas, making it difficult to recruit and retain a sufficient labor supply in other parts of the country.

Before examining some of the current efforts to improve the U.S. health care system, let's examine what to expect as baby boomers age and place increased demands on the industry.

Impact of the Baby Boomer Population

The elderly population in the United States is growing rapidly due to the aging of the baby boomer population—the 78 million people born between 1946 and 1964. Here are some things to consider about this large population:

- Every 8 seconds another baby boomer turns 50 years of age; the over-65 population will almost double by 2030.
- The first baby boomer reached 64 in 2010; it will take another 21 years for the last one to reach that milestone.
- When compared with previous generations, baby boomers have higher education levels, use more online resources, and are more directly involved in their health care.
- Almost 20% of baby boomers are minorities, requiring health care workers to pay more attention to cultural differences.
- Baby boomers possess 75% of the nation's disposable income but worry about covering their health care and retirement expenses.
- Thanks to joint replacements and other medical advancements, baby boomers are more physically active than seniors in the past and suffer from fewer disabilities.

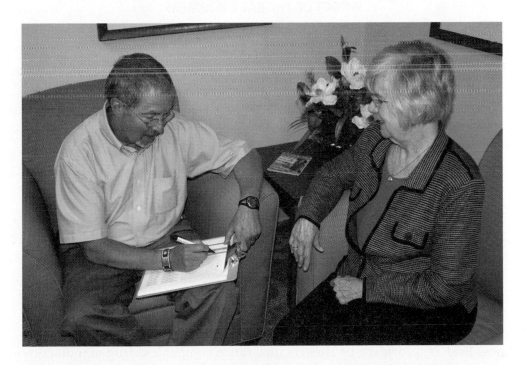

Figure 1-2 ■ Members of the baby boomer population completing paperwork

- Seventy percent of baby boomers subscribe to **alternative medicine** (using healing arts which are not part of traditional medical practice in the United States) or **complementary medicine** (combining alternative medical approaches with traditional medical practices) such as massage therapy, chiropractic care, meditation, and acupuncture.

Efforts are already underway to prepare for the impact of this large patient population. New medicines, monitoring equipment, and surgical techniques are in development. With new technology, seniors will be able to monitor more of their conditions from home and communicate remotely with physicians and specialists. Hospitals are remodeling to offer the more personalized care and the convenience that baby boomers expect, including more private rooms with sound-reduction materials and in-room computers for patient use.

These are just a few examples of how health care providers are preparing for the arrival of this large population of elderly patients but much more needs to be done to improve the nation's health care system for all patients.

CONSIDER THIS

IMPACT OF THE BABY BOOMERS

Baby boomers are predicted to have an unprecedented long-term impact on the health care industry, consuming far more medical services than any elderly population in the past. Baby boomers will live longer than their predecessors. In fact, half of all of the people who have ever lived to age 65 are alive today. By the year 2030, six out of 10 seniors will have at least one chronic condition, one out of three will be considered **obese** (weighing more than 20% over a person's ideal weight), one out of four will have diabetes, and one out of two will be living with arthritis. More than 25% of the total health care spending for each patient occurs in the final years of his or her life. By the year 2030, four out of 10 adult visits to doctors' offices will be conducted by baby boomers, 55 million lab tests per year will be needed for diabetic seniors, eight times more knee replacements will be performed than today, and four million more emergency department visits will be logged than today.

Improving the Nation's Health Care System

As large numbers of baby boomers interact more frequently with the health care system, they will likely become even more engaged in improvement efforts. In doing so, they will join the increasing number of lawmakers, employers, business leaders, providers, consumers, insurance companies, drug manufacturers, and other groups calling for health care reform. There's no question that the United States has one of the best health care systems in the world but the

United States lags behind other countries in **life expectancy** (the number of years of life remaining at any given age), **infant mortality rate** (number of infants that die during the first year of life), preventive care, and other common measures of health and well-being. Studies indicate that as much as one-third of what is spent on health care isn't really necessary. Most everyone agrees there are ample opportunities for improvement and many are calling for extensive reform.

Health Care Reform

As health care costs continue to rise and millions of Americans remain uninsured or underinsured, people agree that something must be done to control costs and increase access to health care. But there is little agreement about how to improve things. After many months of heated debate and negotiation, the Patient Protection and Affordable Care Act (PPACA) became law in 2010. However, many stakeholders don't support the law and are taking steps to change it or overturn it. Some feel the law went too far in involving the government in the health insurance industry while others feel the law didn't go far enough to control costs and overhaul the health care system.

Efforts to improve the nation's health insurance system focus on issues such as the following:

- *Eligibility:* Should people who already have medical problems be eligible for health insurance?
- *Dependents:* What is the maximum age that children can be covered on their parent's insurance policy?
- *Prevention:* Should insurance companies be required to cover preventive services and, if so, which ones?
- *Benefit limitations:* What limits should be placed on annual and lifetime insurance benefits?
- *Cancellation:* Under what conditions should an insurance company be allowed to cancel a policy?
- *Waiting period:* How long should a person have to wait for new health insurance coverage to take effect?

Several terms that are frequently used relate to the effect of health care reform on individual patients. It's important to be familiar with these terms so you can "speak the language" of health care reform:

Preexisting condition: when the patient has a medical condition prior to applying for health insurance

Individual mandate: a requirement that everyone must have health insurance coverage or pay a penalty

Out-of-pocket expense: costs that patients have to pay themselves

Donut hole: the gap in insurance coverage for prescription drugs that Medicare patients must pay themselves

Defensive medicine: when doctors order tests and treatments for patients to avoid potential lawsuits

Much of the controversy surrounding health care reform centers on how to pay for health care services. The following terms represent some of the options under discussion:

Managed care: a health care system where primary care doctors act as gatekeepers to manage each patient's care in a cost-effective manner

Capitation: when a doctor, hospital, or clinic receives a fixed amount of money per person to provide health care services for that person

Single-payer system: when the government collects taxes for health care from all citizens and then uses the collected money to pay for the citizens' health care services

Universal health care: an organized health care system where everyone has health insurance coverage

New types of health care organizations are under discussion as part of health care reform. **Health care exchanges** are open marketplaces where buyers and sellers of health insurance come together to help consumers compare and shop for coverage. **Medical homes** are organizations that deliver primary care (including acute, chronic, and preventative services) through a comprehensive team approach that ensures quality outcomes.

Another concept—**accountable care organizations**—is growing rapidly as one of the most talked-about strategies in health care reform. ACOs are networks of hospitals and doctors that work together and share responsibility and **accountability** (willing to accept responsibility and the consequences of one's actions) for managing all health care services for at least 5,000 Medicare patients over a minimum of three years. Primary care doctors, specialists, home health companies, rehab centers, and hospitals collaborate to eliminate duplicative tests and procedures, focus on prevention, manage diseases, share medical information, care for patients in the least-expensive settings (outpatient clinics and doctor's offices as opposed to emergency departments), and reduce medical **errors** (things done incorrectly through ignorance or carelessness.). Under the new plan, accountable care organizations would receive financial incentives to reduce costs while achieving quality outcomes— thereby getting paid more to keep their patients healthy and out of the hospital. ACOs that fail to meet performance and financial expectations could face financial penalties. This plan is quite different from the current fee-for-service approach in which providers receive payment based on the number and types of diagnostic tests and treatments they order and perform. The advent of ACOs is already having an impact on the U.S. health care system as providers rush to form or enlarge their networks and adopt strategies to become integrated systems. Patient satisfaction is also expected to play a major role in health care reform.

THINK ABOUT IT

HEALTH CARE REFORM

Where do you stand on efforts to reform the nation's health care system? Since you work in health care, people will assume that you know what's going on and will have thoughts to share. Think about questions such as these:

- What role, if any, should the government play in health care and health care reform?
- Should taxpayers cover the cost of health care for people who can't afford it?
- What changes, if any, should be made to Medicare and Medicaid to reduce the cost to taxpayers?
- Should people be required to have health insurance or pay a penalty if they don't want the insurance, believe they don't need it, or can't afford it?
- Should employers have to provide health insurance for their employees or pay a penalty?

As stakeholders consider options to reform Medicare and Medicaid, revisit medical **malpractice** (negligence, failure to meet the standard of care or conduct prescribed by a profession) laws to reduce defensive medicine, and create new ways for people to purchase affordable health insurance, there are several other efforts underway to improve the U.S. health care system. As you prepare for your role in health care, it's important to be aware of these trends and issues.

Quality Improvement

Improving the quality of health care services to achieve better patient outcomes has always been a top priority in health care, but it's even more important today when the goal is to "do more, with less, and get better results." By closely monitoring patient outcomes, providers can make sure that quality doesn't drop as cost cutting and health care reform efforts kick in.

One of the most important steps in improving quality is closely examining the **process** by which work gets done. Examining work processes is especially important when something goes wrong. In health care, this is called **continuous quality improvement (CQI)**—the regular use of methods and tools to identify, prevent, and reduce the impact of process failures. By studying the process, you can determine if there's a better way to do things. When something goes wrong, it's important to figure out what happened and implement a better process to prevent the occurrence from happening again. It's also critical to make sure that quality improvement efforts in your department don't result in a negative impact on other departments.

When doing CQI projects, you must remain focused on what you're trying to do. Ask yourself these questions: (1) What are we trying to accomplish?

(2) How will we know if we are successful? (3) What options do we have and which ones might work best?

Quality improvement (QI) goals include:

- Eliminating **adverse effects** (unfavorable or harmful outcomes) such as patient falls and bed sores
- Reducing waste and unnecessary expense such as duplicating blood tests or keeping patients in the hospital longer than necessary
- Avoiding costly hospital **readmissions** (quick returns to the hospital after discharge)
- Preventing undesirable patient outcomes such as hospital-acquired infections or medication overdoses

Of course, quality improvement is much more than just preventing things from going wrong. Hospitals and other health care providers use quality improvement approaches such as PDSA to figure out how to make things that are working well work even better.

Plan: creating a plan or a test to see how a different approach would work

Do: implementing the plan to see what happens

Study: reviewing the results to determine what was learned

Act: taking action based on what was learned

When using the PDSA approach, you might have to go through the four-step cycle several times before you get the results you're seeking. Using **metrics** (a set of measurements that quantify results) is the key. In most CQI projects, you must be able to measure things to know if your approach was an improvement or not. You gather **baseline data** (gathering information before a change begins to better understand the current situation) before you start and compare those statistics with your **outcome data** (information gathered after a change has occurred to examine the impact or results) after you finish to see if there's been any change and, if so, how much.

There are many ways to improve quality in health care, not the least of which relates to **staffing levels** (the number of people with certain qualifications who are assigned to work at a given time). For example, studies have shown that having an adequate supply of registered nurses on a patient care unit is directly related to the quality of care those patients receive. When hospitals, clinics, and doctors' offices cut back on staff, there's a greater likelihood that quality and patient care will suffer. It's important for health care providers to maintain sufficient staffing levels while monitoring their labor costs. Staffing models that give bedside nurses and other caregivers more responsibility for quality and safety lead to better patient outcomes.

Health care providers and other stakeholders use a lengthy list of indicators to measure quality. Here are just a few examples:

- *Aspirin at arrival:* The percent of heart attack patients who are given aspirin upon arrival at the hospital (Patients should receive aspirin within 24 hours before or after they arrive at the hospital to reduce the potential for blood clots.)
- *Oxygenation assessment:* The percent of patients with pneumonia who have their blood/oxygen level measured (Pneumonia reduces the amount of oxygen in the patient's blood.)
- *Surgical infection prevention care:* The percentage of surgery patients who receive an antibiotic within one hour before surgically cutting the skin (Antibiotics reduce the risk of infection; however, antibiotics must be used with caution to avoid risks associated with multi-resistant organisms.)

Six Sigma, a strategy that incorporates data and statistical analysis to measure and improve a company's operational performance, has been used successfully for many years in the manufacturing industry. This strategy is now helping health care organizations improve their existing processes and develop new processes to meet quality goals. When Six Sigma's lean concepts are applied throughout an entire organization, they can improve work flow, productivity, and the timely delivery of services while reducing waste and costs. Teams from different departments work together to examine each step in the process. When the process breaks down, they look for the **root cause** of the problem (the factor that, when fixed, will solve a problem and prevent it from happening again) instead of just blaming someone. By openly sharing information across departments, Six Sigma teams try to develop a perfect process in which each step creates value for the customer.

Quality improvement projects are often closely aligned with efforts to improve patient safety. Let's take a closer look at patient safety issues.

RECENT DEVELOPMENTS

GREEN MOVEMENT

Health care organizations are joining the green movement, incorporating recycling and waste management programs. New buildings are designed with energy efficiency in mind using recycled and natural building materials, natural lighting, and energy-efficient windows and utility plants. Retired computers and electronics are scrubbed clean of private information and disposed of safely. Environmentally friendly construction materials are helping to reduce the risk of bacterial infections. Building materials and landscaping plants are sourced locally to reduce transportation costs and fuel use. Sensors on public toilets and lavatories are conserving water.

Patient Safety

Health care is one of the most complex industries on Earth. Hundreds of medical miracles occur every day as dedicated, hard-working health care professionals do their best to care for patients. But as you've already learned, the health care system is not perfect. Consider the following sober statistics:

- Death by medical **mistakes** is the third leading cause of death in the United States.
- Each year about one million people are injured and 98,000 die as a result of medical errors.
- Two million patients per year suffer hospital-acquired infections.
- Although the United States spends the most money on health care among developed nations, it scores more poorly than most on quality indicators.

Improving patient safety requires a heightened awareness of errors and mistakes and a culture that encourages nurses and other health care workers to speak up when they see mistakes about to occur. Nurses and other health professionals who interact frequently with their patients get to know their patients quite well. These caregivers must feel **empowered** (to give authority, to enable or permit) to question things when they don't seem right. For example, a nurse might question the doctor's order to give a patient a certain drug if the nurse believes the drug might cause a complication with other drugs the patient is taking. Or a medical assistant might notice that a busy doctor forgot to properly wash his or her hands when moving from a patient with the flu to the next patient who is seeking prenatal care.

Speaking up when you spot something that doesn't seem right may require some courage on your part, especially when questioning someone with more authority, but it's absolutely essential in protecting the patient's safety. Ask yourself this—if you were about to make a mistake that could potentially harm a patient, wouldn't you want someone to speak up, even if it might cause you some embarrassment? Health care professionals always put what is best for their patients ahead of what is best for them. Be on the lookout for potential mistakes and errors and never hesitate to speak up.

A primary goal of patient safety is preventing a **sentinel event**—an unexpected occurrence involving death or serious physical or psychological injury, or the risk thereof with "serious injuries" including the loss of a limb or its function. Each accredited hospital or health care organization is required to define a sentinel event for their purposes and to have a plan in place to identify, report, and manage these kinds of events. Once the event has been reported, the circumstances can be studied and processes can be put into place to prevent the occurrence from happening again.

Each year, National Patient Safety Goals put out by the Joint Commission provide a series of specific actions that accredited organizations are expected to implement to prevent medical errors. Here are a few examples:

- Identify patients correctly; use at least two ways to identify patients (such as the patient's name and date of birth) to make sure that all patients get the medicine, treatment, and blood type meant for them.

- Use medicines safely; label all medicines that are not already labeled (such as medicine in syringes, cups, and basins); take extra care with patients who take blood thinners.
- Prevent infection; use hand-cleaning guidelines to prevent difficult-to-treat infections; use proven guidelines to prevent infection of the blood from central lines (tubes inserted into a patient's vein to administer medications or fluids); use safe practices to treat the part of the body where surgery was done.
- Improve staff communication; quickly get important test results to the right staff person.

As mentioned previously, having an adequate supply of registered nurses on hand is crucial to ensuring quality care and patient safety but shifting trends in the supply and demand of health care workers is causing serious concerns.

Workforce Supply and Demand

Much has been already been said about the impact of the baby boomer population on the health care industry. But the baby boomers' increasing demand for health care services is only part of the problem. Millions of baby boomers work in health care, serving as doctors, nurses, and other

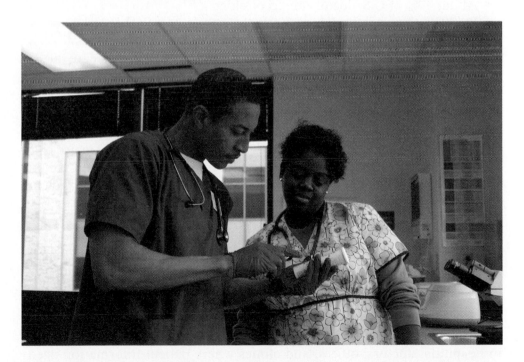

Figure 1-3 ■ Double-checking sample labeling to ensure patient safety

health care workers. As they age, they will retire from their health care jobs in large numbers. These rising retirement rates could lead to major labor shortages during the same period of time when baby boomers themselves are increasing the demand for health care services.

Consider the following:

- About one-third of all registered nurses are currently 50 years of age or older.
- About 55% of RNs plan to retire in the next 10 years.
- By 2020 there will be a shortage of one million nurses in the United States.
- While 50% of nurses currently work in hospitals, the demand in other care settings is growing.
- The number of new RNs graduating from college is not sufficient to replace all of the retiring nurses.
- To meet the demand, new nursing graduates would have to increase by 90% a year.
- As the demand for RNs increases worldwide, there will be fewer foreign-trained nurses to work in the United States.

Labor shortages are also predicted for other types of health care professionals, including doctors.

- About 40% of U.S. doctors are 55 or older.
- By 2020, there will be at least 100,000 fewer doctors in the workplace than today.
- There's already a shortage of **geriatric** (specializing in health care for elderly patients) doctors and the supply is declining.
- Even if the number stabilizes, there will be a shortage of 20,000 geriatricians by 2015.

When you match these labor forecasts with the expected demands of the baby boomer population, you can easily understand some of the major challenges facing the U.S. health care system. Keep this sobering fact in mind—these forecasts do not include the additional patients who will be showing up for health care services if and when health care reform expands access to millions of additional patients.

There is some good news in all of this. Advancements in technology are improving patient care, quality, and safety in ways we couldn't even imagine just a few years ago. Let's take a look at just one of the ways technology is improving the nation's health care system—electronic medical records.

Electronic Medical Records

Electronic medical records (EMRs) are becoming increasingly common in hospitals, doctors' offices, and clinics where patient information needs to be shared quickly and frequently among providers at several different locations. When patients move among doctors' offices, specialists, clinics, and hospitals, their medical information needs to move with them. This is best accomplished by using technology. When providers can access comprehensive, up-to-date information on each patient, the quality and continuity of care increases and the cost associated with unnecessary duplication of blood tests and radiographs, for example, decreases. EMRs offer several other advantages. They:

- *Save paper and space.* Instead of keeping paper files on patients, health care providers keep patients' medical records in computer files, which saves space and reduces storage costs.
- *Enhance coordination.* All members of the patient's health care team, regardless of their locations, have access to the same medical information. They can see what other team members are doing to care for the patient as they develop their own treatment plans.
- *Improve quality.* When patients are being seen by several specialists at the same time, there's a risk that one doctor might prescribe a drug that isn't compatible with the drugs prescribed by another doctor. With EMRs, each doctor can see what the other doctors are prescribing. This is just one example of quality improvement via EMRs.
- *Reduce delays.* When doctors need to review a patient's paper medical records, the pages must be copied, mailed, faxed, or scanned and emailed to other locations. This takes time and can delay the patient's tests and treatments. But when doctors use technology to gain immediate access to records, tests and treatments can begin much sooner. This is especially important in emergency situations when response time is critical.
- *Ensure* **legibility** *(hand-writing that can be read and accurately interpreted by another person).* Hand-written doctors' orders and treatment notes can be difficult to read, sometimes leading to confusion or mistakes. When orders and treatment notes are typed into an electronic record, illegible hand-writing is no longer a concern although typos can still occur.

As with most technologic advancements, there are also some disadvantages to EMRs:

- *Training time and anxiety.* Doctors, nurses, and other health care workers must be trained to use EMRs. Undergoing training and mastering new skills take time, which can cause a backlog in caring for patients until the staff is up to speed with the new technology. Some people, especially older workers, may resist having to learn new skills, which can lead to anxiety and frustration.
- *System incompatability.* There is no universal EMR, and different systems won't always interact with one another. This is one reason why health care providers are joining networks so that all members within the network can use the same electronic systems.

• *Security concerns.* Having medical information stored on computers raises concerns about potential security issues and the accidental release of private information. Staff must follow strict security measures when storing, transmitting, and transporting medical records electronically to avoid a **breach** (a break, failure, or interruption) in **confidentiality** (maintaining the privacy of certain matters).

In spite of the disadvantages, the push is on to convert to electronic medical records. Doing so will require time and money, but the long-term benefits most likely will be worth the investment.

What could be more exciting than watching new technology emerge in health care? You'll need to know what types of new technology are on the drawing board for your profession and how that technology will affect your patients and your work. Most of the computer software, drugs, devices, and medical procedures that will be routine tomorrow haven't even been developed yet. Maybe you will play a role in discovering a medical breakthrough at some point in your career.

The Big Picture and Where You Fit In

Having taken a step back to look at the big picture of the health care industry and its trends and issues, it should be obvious by now that you have your work cut out for you. You must view the health care industry from the service side and the business side and try to keep both in balance.

You'll wear at least three different hats—as a patient, taxpayer, and health care professional. Each time you change a hat, your **perspective** (the manner in which a person views something) will change along with it. Some of your perspectives might conflict with the others. Here are a few examples:

What's best for you as a patient might not be what's best for you as a taxpayer. As a patient you want the very best health care that money can buy, no matter what the cost, but as a taxpayer you know that resources to fund medical care are limited.

What's best for you as a health care professional might not be what's best for you as a patient. As a health care professional you want to leave work on time to get on with your busy personal life but as a patient you want your caregiver to stay as late as necessary to finish your procedure before handing you off to the next shift.

What's best for you as a taxpayer might not be what's best for you as a health care professional. As a taxpayer you want to reduce the cost of health care to avoid tax increases but as a health care professional you want the government to fund medical research to help develop new treatments and cures.

In order to make the best decisions, you must keep all of these perspectives in mind as you move through the day. Always try to see things through the eyes of your patients because when you're at work wearing your health care professional hat, your patients must always come first.

For More Information

The Health Care Industry
American Hospital Association
www.aha.org
312-422-3000

Health Care Reform
www.healthcare.gov
U.S. Department of Health
and Human Services
877-696-6775

Health Care Labor Forecasts
Bureau of Labor Statistics,
U.S. Department of Labor
www.bls.gov
202-691-5200

Baby Boomer Population
www.babyboomers.com

National Patient Safety Goals
www.jointcommission.org/standards

Quality Improvement
Agency for Healthcare Research
and Quality (AHRQ)
U.S. Department of Health
and Human Services
www.ahrq.gov
301-427-1104

Six Sigma
www.isixsigma.com

REALITY CHECK

It's time to get real and think about answering the question, What role are you going to play?

Will you be one of those people who just passes through, skipping from job to job and paycheck to paycheck? Or will you take your career seriously and make the most of it? Will you lie, cheat, and steal from your employer or live up to high standards and set a good example for other people?

Some health care workers are like renters and others are like owners. Renters have a short-term outlook. They don't feel a sense of ownership so they avoid investing their time, money, and energy in making improvements. Owners, however, are in it for the long term. They not only invest in improvements but they also take pride in the results.

The future is before you. What you make of it is up to you.

If you're serious about a career in health care and your goal is to be recognized as a health care professional then keep reading. It's time to learn more about what's going to be expected of you. The remainder of this book provides a roadmap to success.

Key Points

- Remember that soft skills are just as important as hard skills in achieving success at work.
- Keep up-to-date with the business side of health care and where it appears to be headed.
- Monitor current trends and issues so you can discuss them intelligently with other people.
- Be on the lookout for new technology and how it might impact your patients and your work.
- Apply the PDSA approach and statistical measurements to improve the quality of care.
- Monitor National Patient Safety Goals and avoid potential mistakes and errors.
- Speak up and question the actions of others when something doesn't seem quite right.
- Learn as much as you can about caring for geriatric patients.
- Embrace new technology, such as electronic medical records, and the benefits it provides.
- Think about the different hats you wear and always put your patients first.
- Consider what role *you* want to play in health care and keep learning.

Learning Activities

Using information from Chapter One:
- Answer the Chapter Review Questions.
- Respond to the What If? Scenarios.
- Complete Chapter One activities on the website.

Chapter Review Questions

Using information presented in Chapter One, answer each of the following questions:
1. List four benefits of working in the health care industry.

2. Define *soft skills* and *hard skills*, explain the difference, and discuss why both are important.

3. List two reasons why it's important for health care professionals to know about current trends and issues in the health care industry.

4. List three reasons why health care is expensive and the cost continues to rise.

5. Identify four ways that the baby boomer population will impact the health care industry.

6. Identify and discuss two controversial issues associated with health care reform.

7. Define *continuous quality improvement* and list two quality improvement goals.

8. Define *sentinel event* and explain the connection between sentinel events and patient safety.

9. Identify two trends in the supply and demand of health care workers.

10. List two advantages and disadvantages of electronic medical records.

What If? Scenarios

Think about what you would do in the following situations and record your answers.

1. You need to analyze data on 100 patients and issue a report. The database you'll be using includes Social Security numbers, addresses, and sensitive medical information about each patient. The deadline to submit your report is just a week away and you have several other things to do between now and then. If you download the data on a flash drive (a small, 2- to 3-inch portable data device that stores several gigabytes of information) you can work on the project at home over the weekend and avoid having to come back into the office.

2. You're the leader of a team that includes a new employee. He has years of experience working in another hospital and knows more than the rest of the team about operating the new high tech equipment just installed in your department. When you ask him to show his coworkers how to use the new equipment, he refuses by saying, "I wasn't hired to be a teacher." He mostly keeps to himself and doesn't get along very well with other team members. You're beginning to wonder which is more important—hard skills or soft skills.

3. You've been invited to participate on a conference panel next month to discuss the impact of health care reform on your profession. You really want to accept the invitation but you don't feel prepared. You've heard just enough about health care reform on TV to know it's a controversial topic. You read a newspaper article stating that health insurance is changing. And you overheard a heated conversation last week between your father and uncle arguing about taxes, Medicare, and something called an individual mandate.

4. Your neighbor has paid you a visit, very upset about the bill he just received for having some blood tests run at a local clinic. He said the cost this year was 25% higher than what he was charged for the same tests a year ago. Since you work in health care, he wants you to explain why the cost has gone up so much and what, if anything, is being done to reduce the expense.

5. The outpatient surgery center where you work just experienced a sentinel event, resulting in serious harm to one of the patients. It was a complicated case and no one knows what exactly what went wrong. The surgeons and staff are highly concerned that the same thing might happen again unless the cause can be identified and fixed.

6. A doctor on your unit just ordered a drug for one of your patients. You're pretty sure that the drug she ordered will cause a serious complication with another drug ordered by another doctor just yesterday. You are new on the unit and not sure if you should speak up or not.

7. You really need the day off tomorrow but forgot to take your name off the schedule. You could call in sick but your absence would cause the staffing level to drop below what's safe for the patients.

Your Work Ethic and Performance

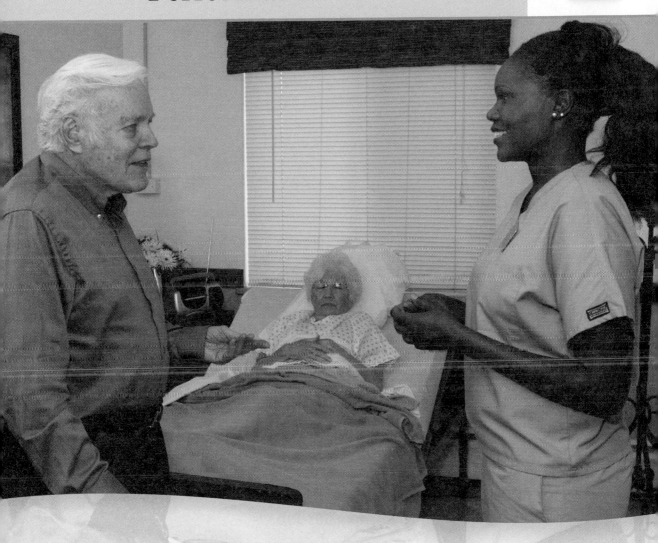

"A pessimist sees the difficulty in every opportunity. An optimist sees the opportunity in every difficulty."

Winston Churchill,
British prime minister, 1874–1965

CHAPTER OBJECTIVES

Having completed this chapter, you will be able to:

- Define *interdependence* and *systems perspective* and explain their importance in health care.

- Explain why it's important to be "present in the moment" at work.

- Define *critical thinking* and list three things that critical thinkers do to make good decisions.

- List five factors that demonstrate a strong work ethic.

- Describe the attitudinal differences between optimists and pessimists.

- Discuss the importance of confidentiality and HIPAA.

- Identify how competence and scope of practice impact quality of care.

- List two things you should do when representing your employer.

- Explain the purpose of performance evaluations and list three ways to prepare for one.

- Differentiate between objective and subjective evaluation criteria.

KEY TERMS

compliance	front-line workers	peers	sexual harassment
conflict of interest	goals	performance	social networking
constructive	HIPAA	evaluations	sites
criticism	HITECH	pessimists	stagnant
contingency plans	hostile workplace	probationary period	subjective
corporate mission	impaired	problem solving	subordinates
corporate values	insubordination	punctual	systematic
corrective action	intentional	rational	systems perspective
critical thinking	interdependence	reasoning	unethical
diligent	objective	reimbursement	up-code
discretion	optimists	reliability	whistle blower
dismissal	organizational chart	responsibility	360-degree feedback
fraudulent		self-awareness	

Making a Commitment to Your Job

No job is insignificant and no worker is unimportant in health care. Most people are familiar with the critical roles that doctors, nurses, and pharmacists play in health care, but patients and the general public may not be as familiar with the roles of other caregivers such as medical assistants, nuclear medicine technologists, occupational therapists, electroneurodiagnostic (END) technologists, and sonographers, to name just a few. People who work behind the scenes may be even less known to patients and the public. This includes instrument technicians, biomedical engineers, research assistants, and medical coders whose roles are also vital. When you add chefs, security officers, lawyers, and maintenance workers, large urban hospitals and medical centers employ so many different types of workers they begin to resemble small towns. Depending on how you add them up, there are several hundred different jobs in health care organizations.

If your job involves direct patient care, it should be obvious that professionalism is important. The same holds true with jobs in which workers interact with visitors, guests, and vendors or function in support roles behind the scenes. Examples include customer service agents, telephone operators, purchasing agents, billing clerks, insurance processors, and medical secretaries. Professionalism is important in all jobs. Consider what might happen in the following situations:

- What if phlebotomists confuse blood samples and label them incorrectly?
- What if clerical workers misspell medical terms on patient records?
- What if housekeepers don't dispose of soiled linen properly?
- What if radiographers position patients incorrectly and have to repeat imaging exams?

It should be obvious that professionalism is vital in every job. Each job exists for a reason, and performing the job well requires making a commitment to your job and taking a professional approach to your work.

Interdependence

As mentioned previously, no matter what your job may involve you must be able to view the big picture and know where and how you fit in. Having examined the health care industry in general, let's focus more closely on your job and how it connects with the roles of other workers. This starts with developing a **systems perspective**—stepping back to view an entire process to see how each component connects with the others. No one in health care works alone; everyone's work is interconnected. This reliance on one another is called **interdependence** and without it the work flow breaks down.

Think about your role and responsibilities:

- How do your responsibilities connect with those of other workers?
- Which other workers do you have to depend on to get your work done?
- Which other workers have to depend on you to get their work done?
- Where do the patients fit into this picture?

Most companies have an **organizational chart**—an illustration showing the components of a company and how they fit together. Typical organizational charts include the hierarchy of the company—people and work units arranged by rank, in other words, "who" reports "to whom." Large companies have detailed illustrations showing the flow of work processes within and across departments. Regardless of the size and structure of the company, there's always one common thread—all departments and employees must work together and depend on one another to get the work done and done well.

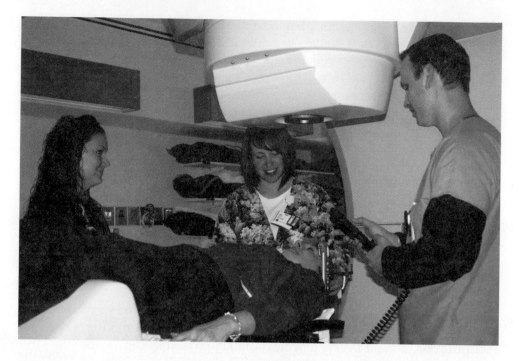

Figure 2-1 ■ Teamwork in positioning a patient for treatment

From a systems perspective, ask yourself what would happen if you:

- Don't show up for work on time and fail to notify someone?
- Get sloppy and make an error?
- Appear for work **impaired** by alcohol or an illegal or prescription drug?

How would these behaviors affect other workers who are counting on you? If you fail to commit to your job, you won't be there for long. You may be able to hide incompetence, sloppiness, and indifference for a little while but eventually poor performance will catch up with you. What's worse, someone could be harmed by your lack of commitment and professionalism in the meantime.

Self-Awareness

One of the challenges of working in a busy environment is avoiding distractions and paying attention to what's going on around you. This requires a certain degree of **self-awareness**—understanding where you are, what you're doing, and why you're doing it. This involves the concept of being "present in the moment." When you are present in the moment you can filter out distractions and concentrate on what's in front of you at any given time. This ability to focus is absolutely critical in avoiding mistakes and errors. It's important to stop and think before you act. Everything that you say and do should be **intentional**. This means thinking things through and doing and saying things on purpose rather than just quickly reacting to whatever situation occurs.

When you are at work you need to filter out distractions from your personal life, which is easier said than done. Family conflicts, an argument with your spouse, bill collectors finding you at work, children left unsupervised, legal issues and court dates, and your own medical concerns are just a few examples of situations in your personal life that can cause distractions at work. Let's face it—you're just one person and it's not easy to keep everything in balance. Concentrating on the task at hand when there's so much else going on around you can be quite a challenge, but it's something you must work hard to achieve.

One of the best ways to reduce distractions at work is to avoid becoming a distraction yourself. You aren't there to sell things, convince coworkers to adopt your political or religious beliefs, plan social gatherings, spread gossip, text friends, visit **social networking sites** (Internet places for people to publish and share personal information), shop online, wager bets, or collect donations for your favorite charity. You are there to work, not to advance your personal agenda. Save distracting activities such as these for after work hours.

Working in health care is stressful. Each day that you come to work you'll be faced with a variety of decisions to make and problems to solve. The facts and data that you've learned in school will certainly help but making good decisions and finding workable solutions requires the ability to fully understand, explore, question, and apply the information you've learned in the past. When it comes to patient care, there isn't always just one right way to do things. You have to think through each situation, decide on a strategy, test it, observe the results, and adjust accordingly. This is where critical thinking becomes a valuable skill.

Critical Thinking

What is critical thinking? **Critical thinking** is using **reasoning** (forming conclusions based on coherent and logical thinking) and evidence to make decisions about what to do or believe without being influenced by emotions. By using critical thinking skills and a step-by-step **systematic** approach (a methodical procedure or plan) to decision making, you can reduce your stress and find effective solutions to almost any problem. When you think critically, you:

- Look at things from a **rational** (based on reason; logical) and practical perspective
- Ask essential questions to get to the heart of the matter
- Identify and analyze relevant information and evidence

- Differentiate among facts, opinions, and personal feelings
- Think with an open mind and question assumptions
- Exercise caution in drawing conclusions
- Test conclusions against relevant standards

When faced with a problem, critical thinking skills can help you:

- Avoid jumping to conclusions
- Identify and clarify the problem
- Gather as much information as you can
- Examine the evidence you've found
- Identify options to solve the problem
- Decide which option would work best
- Implement your solution
- Evaluate the results

There's almost always a good solution to every problem but you may have to invest some time and energy to find it.

Effective **problem solving** and critical thinking skills are mandatory for a well-orchestrated personal and professional life. Interpreting the small print in credit card agreements, creating a budget for your family, comparing options for car insurance, and figuring out how to resolve an argument with a friend are just a few examples of when critical thinking skills can help you personally. Selecting the appropriate equipment settings, revising a patient's treatment plan, interpreting blood test results, and deciding whether to apply for a promotion are just a few examples of how critical thinking skills can help guide you in the right direction professionally. Developing critical thinking and problem-solving skills takes time but it is well worth the investment. The more you use your skills, the better they will become.

Developing a Strong Work Ethic

Ask employers what characteristic is most important in a good employee and the majority will respond "a strong work ethic." Having a strong work ethic means positioning your job as a high priority in your life and making sound decisions about how you approach your work. Employees with a strong work ethic:

- Stay focused and leave their personal problems at home
- Apply themselves to the task at hand
- Get their work done right the first time
- Exercise self-discipline and self-control
- Know what management expects of them and apply themselves as needed
- Don't wait to be told what to do
- Demonstrate a positive attitude and enthusiasm for their work

Let's examine some additional factors that describe a strong work ethic.

Attendance and Punctuality

It's nearly impossible to demonstrate a commitment to your job without being there. Performing the duties of your job requires showing up for work every day and being **punctual** (arriving for work on time). Poor attendance usually results in other people having to cover for you when you aren't there. How would you feel if your coworkers called in sick frequently, leaving you to do your work plus their work? How would your coworkers feel if your attendance leaves a lot to be desired? Many health care organizations are already lean on staffing and can't afford to have people absent on a regular basis. When people are counting on you, it's important to be there and to arrive on time.

When you arrive late for work:

- The patient's diagnosis, treatment, surgery, or discharge from the hospital might be delayed.
- Necessary supplies might not get delivered on time.
- Paperwork might get filed too late to meet a deadline.
- Other people might have to work late to catch up.

Remember how the roles of health care workers are interconnected? You may think arriving late won't cause a problem for your work group, but what complications might you be causing other people?

Most everyone must miss work or arrive late on occasion, but when poor attendance or lack of punctuality becomes a habit, it may result in a performance issue leading to **corrective action** (steps taken to overcome a job performance problem) or **dismissal** (involuntary termination from a job).

What steps can you take to ensure good attendance and punctuality?

- Make a commitment to show up for work every day and arrive on time.
- When your shift starts, make sure you are in the area and ready to go.
- Have **contingency plans** (backup plans in case the original plans don't work) to cover situations when your children or spouse gets sick or when your transportation becomes unreliable.
- Protect your health and safety to keep from getting sick or injured.
- Eat well, get plenty of sleep, and consider getting a flu shot.

Allow some extra time at the end of your shift in case you get held over. Never leave a patient or coworker "hanging" by rushing out the door the minute your shift ends. Make sure there's a smooth transition between shifts and don't leave your work for other people to finish up. Remember interdependence? Other people are counting on you to arrive on time and get your part of the work done.

Reliability and Accountability

Reliability (can be counted upon; trustworthy) and accountability are key factors in a strong work ethic. If reliable people agree to do something, their coworkers know they will follow through. Following through on commitments is a big part of the team effort. If you are there for other people when you say you will be, it's more likely they will be there for you when you need them.

People who are accountable accept **responsibility** (a sense of duty binding someone to a course of action) for the consequences of their actions. They "own up" to what they've done and avoid blaming other people. If you make a mistake, admit it and accept full responsibility. Apologize to those who have been inconvenienced. Keep in mind, however, that although it's important to apologize for a mistake it doesn't erase the fact that a mistake was made. Learn from the experience and avoid making the same mistake twice. Your supervisor and coworkers will appreciate your "the buck stops here" attitude.

Follow through on all work assignments for which you are qualified and prepared to perform. If you are given a work assignment for which you are not qualified to perform or not prepared to perform, discuss the situation with your supervisor immediately. Refusal to complete a task as assigned may be construed as **insubordination** and grounds for dismissal.

When serving the needs of patients, it's important to avoid passing judgment or projecting your own personal beliefs on others. If you object to an assignment because it conflicts with your religious beliefs or values, you must discuss these concerns with your supervisor. It's best to resolve issues like these when you first consider a job offer. If you wish to not participate in abortions, sex change operations, end-of-life procedures, or other such activities, many employers will allow you to opt out but this must be discussed ahead of time so that patient care isn't delayed or jeopardized.

Attitude and Enthusiasm

How often have you witnessed another person's behavior and thought to yourself, "What a bad attitude!" For some people, negativity is a way of life. **Pessimists** (people who look on the dark side of things) see the glass as half empty. From their perspective, their situation is always bad and getting worse. They complain about everything and nothing seems to satisfy them. They rarely smile, appear happy, or convey enthusiasm about their work. They spread negativity to everyone around them and undermine morale, teamwork, and a spirit of cooperation.

Optimists (people who look on the bright side of things), on the other hand, display a positive attitude most of the time. They see the glass as half full and approach life with enthusiasm. When they experience things they disagree with, they voice their complaints in a constructive manner. They look for reasons to feel happy and content and they appreciate the small things in life. They tend to smile a lot and convey a friendly and cooperative attitude.

THINK ABOUT IT

OPTIMIST OR PESSIMIST?

- Are you an optimist or a pessimist?
- Do you focus on the positives of a situation or the negatives?
- What effect does your point of view have on your attitude?
- How does your attitude affect your work and your relationships with other people?
- Is negativity holding you back from a job promotion or more fully enjoying your life?
- What can you do to develop a more positive outlook?

Working in health care can really challenge your attitude. People who have worked in health care for several years may feel as if things are getting worse. They may be critical, resentful, and angry about some of the changes they've seen occur. Perhaps cutting staff to reduce costs has resulted in longer work hours, additional duties, and more holiday shifts to cover. Some of the benefits they enjoyed in the past may have been reduced or eliminated to save money. Their job titles and job duties might have been altered as part of a reorganization or merger of companies.

Health care is constantly changing. When workers feel like something of value has been taken away, their attitudes can suffer. It's important to look for the advantages that come with change and avoid focusing on the negatives.

People who are relatively new in their health careers may also face attitudinal challenges. Young workers may become impatient when job promotions and pay raises don't occur quickly enough. They might question long-standing policies and procedures that don't seem relevant any more. Dress code requirements barring visible tattoos, facial piercings, and non-traditional hair colors and styles may cause discontent.

The bottom line is this: no job or place of employment will ever be perfect. Even though companies may work hard to enhance job satisfaction, people will still find things to complain about. That's just human nature. The key to maintaining a positive attitude is to always look for what's good in any situation and remain optimistic that things will get better.

Displaying enthusiasm and a positive attitude is an important part of a professional's work ethic. If you want to excel and advance in your career, a positive attitude is a must. Here are some choices you can make:

- If you are an optimist, make sure your positive attitude is evident at work.
- If you are a pessimist, put some effort into changing your outlook.
- Look for the bright side in any situation and focus on the positives.
- Seize opportunities to feel happy and appreciate the small things in life.
- When you must complain, express your concerns to the appropriate person in a constructive manner.

If you feel "stressed out" get some help right away. Health care workers who don't alleviate their stress run the risk of damaging their health and spreading their stress among coworkers. Smile every chance you get, even when speaking on the telephone. By adopting a positive attitude, you will experience more joy and greater satisfaction in life and your optimism and enthusiasm will spread to those around you.

Competence and Quality of Work

No matter where your job falls within the organization, the quality of your work is extremely important. What does quality mean to you? What does it mean to your employer and your patients? How can you support quality improvement? Let's start with the importance of competency:

- Make sure you are well trained and competent to perform every function of your job.
- Never take a chance and just "wing it."
- Keep your knowledge up-to-date and your skills sharp.
- Learn about the latest procedures, techniques, and new equipment.
- Attend in-service sessions, register for continuing education workshops, and read professional publications in your field.
- Don't hesitate to ask questions or request help.

Keep in mind that your education won't end when you graduate from school. Nothing stays **stagnant** (without motion; dull, sluggish) in health care. As a professional, it's your responsibility to continue learning, strengthen your skills, and improve the quality of your work.

Perhaps you've heard the saying, "Quality is in the details." This means paying attention to even the smallest things because making a small mistake or overlooking a minor detail can have a big impact on quality. Stocking items on the wrong shelf, misfiling a patient's record, losing a phone number, miscalculating a bill, or missing an important meeting can all negatively affect quality. Each day brings many opportunities for details to fall through the cracks. Being **diligent** (careful in one's work) about quality will help prevent these kinds of problems.

Contributing to companywide quality improvement efforts is an important aspect of your work ethic. No one has a better handle on how to improve work processes and quality outcomes than the people who do the work on a daily basis. Management can't improve the company's quality without the help of their **subordinates** (people at a lower rank). Here are some ways you can improve workplace quality:

- When you have a suggestion for quality improvement, submit it to your supervisor.
- When you spot a potential problem, report it.
- If your work unit receives periodic quality-related data, pay attention to the reports and do your best to support improvements.

Sometimes you may be asked to do things that don't fall within your job description. Responding to one of these requests by saying, "That's not my job!" isn't acceptable. Either you should go ahead and perform the task because you are capable and willing to do it or you should refer the matter to the appropriate person and make sure he or she follows through. No task is too menial when working in health care. Consider the following:

- If a patient or visitor becomes ill in the parking lot, offer assistance or send for help.
- If someone looks lost, provide directions; if necessary, guide the person to his or her destination.
- If you notice a spill in a public area, don't wait for a housekeeper to discover it. Clean it up yourself (using standard precautions) or report it to the appropriate person and stay in the area until it's cleaned up to prevent possible injuries.
- If you observe a piece of equipment not working properly or spot a situation that could pose a health or safety hazard, take action. Don't just ignore things and go on about your business.

A commitment to quality requires paying attention to what's going on around you and addressing concerns before they escalate into serious problems.

Compliance

Compliance (acting in accordance with laws and with a company's rules, policies, and procedures) is extremely important. Ignoring a rule, violating a policy, or breaking the law can compromise quality, hurt a patient or coworker, and get you fired from your job. What might happen if employees:

- Don't wear their identification badges at work?
- Share private business matters or confidential patient information?
- Make threats against other employees?
- Attempt to perform duties beyond their scope of practice?

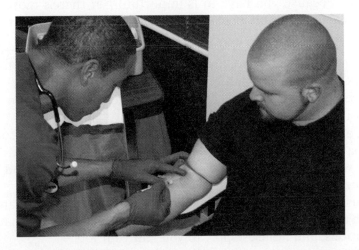

Figure 2-2 ■ Working within scope of practice to perform a phlebotomy procedure

Health care workers must always function within their scope of practice. Performing duties beyond what you're legally permitted to do is highly risky and illegal. Some jobs require a special license to practice. State agencies grant licenses only to people who have met preestablished qualifications and only licensed workers may legally perform the job. Other jobs may require a special certification. State agencies and professional associations certify people who have met certain competency standards. Although noncertified people may legally perform the job, employers may prefer to hire only those workers who possess certification and who are eligible to use the professional title associated with that certification. When a license, certification, or some other special credential is required for your job, make sure you meet those requirements and maintain an active status for that job. In some professions this means completing annual continuing education requirements or periodic competency retesting.

Rules and policies are established for good reasons, and everyone is responsible for complying with them. Health care companies usually have written policies and procedures plus employee handbooks to communicate their expectations. Know where to find these documents and if you don't understand something ask for clarification.

Complying with laws and policies has always been important in health care, but compliance is gaining even more attention these days because the government is stepping up its efforts to identify violators and prosecute them. Some companies have hotlines so employees can report compliance concerns anonymously with no fear of backlash.

Violating a law, regulation, or policy can get you and your employer in serious trouble. You could end up fired, prosecuted, fined, or incarcerated. Your employer could face stiff fines and exclusion from vital government programs such as Medicare or Medicaid. Complying with laws, regulations, and policies because you have to is important but there's more to it than that. Professionals comply because *it's the right thing to do*. Here are some important points:

- Make sure you're aware of and understand all laws, regulations, and policies pertaining to your job.
- Become familiar with medical and legal issues specific to your profession.
- Learn about fire safety procedures and how to protect the security of your patients, coworkers, and company.
- Know what your company expects of you in supporting sound business practices.
- If accused of an illegal activity, claiming that you weren't aware of the law isn't an acceptable legal defense. It's your job to know what laws, regulations, and policies apply to you and your job.
- If you're uncertain about compliance responsibilities, ask for clarification.

A major part of compliance in health care is protecting the confidentiality of patient medical records. The Health Insurance Portability and Accountability Act of 1996 (**HIPAA**) enacted national standards for this purpose. Protecting confidentiality has become even more critical with the advent of electronic medical records. The Health Information Technology for Economic and Clinical Health (**HITECH**) Act was signed into law in February 2009 as part of the American Recovery and Reinvestment Act of 2009 (ARRA). Portions of the HITECH Act address the confidentiality of health information transmitted electronically and strengthen the enforcement and penalties associated with HIPAA rules. Become familiar with what you need to do to comply with HIPAA and the HITECH Act to prevent the inappropriate disclosure of confidential information and avoid potential fines against you and your employer. Also make sure you maintain the confidentiality of financial information and other materials your employer deems private. If you work for more than one health care company at the same time or move from employer to employer, it's important to not share private information among employers.

Some other areas of compliance concerns include safety and environmental precautions, labor laws, retention of records, Medicare billing and **reimbursement** (to pay back or compensate for money spent), licenses and credentials, and **conflict of interest** (an inappropriate relationship between personal interests and official responsibilities).

Examples of illegal or **unethical** (a violation of standards of conduct and moral judgment) behaviors include the following:

- **Fraudulent** (intentional deceit through false information or misrepresentation) billing such as charging for a test or treatment that wasn't performed
- Improperly changing or destroying records
- **Sexual harassment** (unwelcome, sexually-oriented advances or comments)
- Creating a **hostile workplace** (an uncomfortable or unsafe work environment)
- Stealing property

Issues related to sexual harassment can cause major problems at work. Avoid any suggestion of unwelcome sexually-oriented advances or comments that could lead to sexual harassment charges being filed against you. Examples include verbal communication, sending visual and written materials, unwanted touching, sexually explicit texting or postings on social networking sites, or any other actions that have the potential to make another person uncomfortable. Even if you think your actions are harmless, the other person (or someone else present at the time) might see things differently.

If you are the victim of sexual harassment or intimidation, report the incident to your supervisor or another superior immediately. Keep written notes on what you've observed or experienced, including details such as the date, time, place, who was present, what exactly happened, and what you did to follow up. Information such as this will be very important if an investigation takes place.

There are far too many examples of compliance concerns to list them all. Here are some important things to keep in mind:

- Don't modify or destroy patient or financial records without proper authority.
- If your job involves preparing bills for patient procedures, make sure the codes you use to identify specific diagnoses or procedures are accurate; never **up-code** (modifying the classification of a procedure to increase financial reimbursement).
- Always work within your scope of practice.
- Don't accept pay for hours that you did not work.
- Avoid any suggestion of a conflict of interest.
- If your job involves awarding contracts to outside companies, don't accept gifts or free meals in exchange.
- Don't ask a vendor that your company does business with to give you a special discount on a personal purchase.
- Don't refer patients to one of your relatives who just happens to be in the health care business.

Inappropriate Behavior

Inappropriate behavior can result in serious compliance issues. For example, you should never bring a weapon to work or create an environment in which someone else could feel intimidated or unsafe. Avoid verbal threats, nasty letters, or other forms of hostile behavior that may lead to charges of intimidation.

As a professional, you should never knowingly engage in an illegal or unethical act yourself but you might observe someone else doing something suspicious. Or you might feel that you are a victim of sexual harassment or a hostile work environment. If you have a concern about something you see going on at work that might put you, your employer, coworkers, or patients at risk, let your supervisor know or report your concern via a hotline if one is available.

If your supervisor is one of the people involved in the activity, report the matter to your supervisor's boss, a human resources representative, or someone in legal services.

Stay alert! If you find yourself in a situation in which you aren't sure how to proceed, ask yourself some questions. Is what's going on legal and ethical? Is it in the best interests of my employer and patients? How would this look to others outside my organization? Then take action.

You've probably heard the term **whistle blower**—a person who exposes the illegal or unethical practices of another person or of a company. "Blowing the whistle" can be a scary proposition for employees, but the law protects whistle blowers from retribution. In fact, whistle blowers might receive a portion of the fine the government collects when a health care provider is found guilty of Medicare fraud, for example. Here are some first steps if you suspect something illegal is happening in your organization:

- If you suspect someone of illegal or unethical behavior, it's your responsibility to report it.
- Try to resolve your concerns within your organization first. Avoid going to the government or the media unless repeated internal attempts have failed.
- If you've tried your best to report and stop illegal or unethical practices, but have been unsuccessful, you might need to think about finding a job at another company.

CONSIDER THIS

REPORTING ILLEGAL BEHAVIOR

If you know someone is engaged in illegal behavior, it's your responsibility to report it. If you don't report it, you could get in trouble as well. In fact, even if you didn't know the illegal behavior was occurring but you should have known, you can be liable for legal action.

For example, if you observe someone stealing from a patient, report it immediately. If you don't report it and your supervisor finds out that you knew what was going on, you could be disciplined as well as the thief. If your job involves maintaining an inventory of supplies and a coworker gets fired for stealing some of them, you could get in trouble for not noticing the items were missing.

Although you might be tempted to say, "It's none of my business," reporting the illegal behavior of a coworker actually *is* your business.

Representing Your Employer

When you accept a job offer, show up for work, and receive a paycheck, you become a representative of the company. To patients, visitors, guests, and vendors, *you are the company you work for.* Everything you do and say can have an impact on the company's reputation. By accepting employment, you agree not only to follow your company's rules and policies but also to support its mission and values.

Get a copy of your company's **corporate mission** (special duties, functions, or purposes of a company) and **corporate values** (beliefs held in high esteem by a company), review the documents, and think about what you could do to

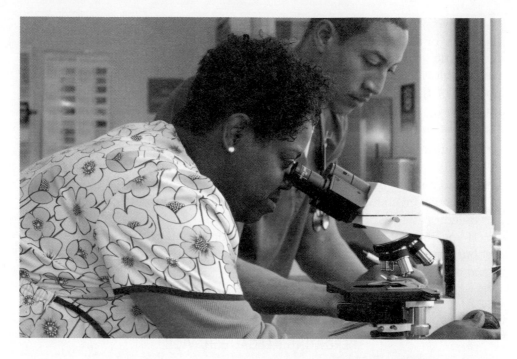

Figure 2-3 ■ Examining a microscopic slide to ensure accuracy

support your employer. Even though you don't own the company, it's important to take an active interest and get involved. Make sure to:

- Learn about the history and structure of your company to discuss it intelligently with other people.
- Read company newsletters and keep up with the latest news and events.
- Participate in your company's social events and sports teams.
- Volunteer to serve on committees and your local speaker's bureau.
- Substitute words such as *we* and *us* for *they* and *them*. For example, instead of saying, "They told us they are going to open a new clinic next year," it would be better to say, "We are opening our new clinic next year."

Take some pride and ownership in the company you work for. It's part of being a professional.

Regardless of what job you have, your appearance, attitudes, and behaviors reflect the company you work for. **Front-line workers** such as nurses, medical assistants, housekeepers, patient transporters, and cafeteria workers have some of the greatest influence on their company's reputation because they have the most frequent contact with patients, visitors, and guests. What might happen if you publicly criticize your employer, complain about a company policy, or question how a physician treated a patient? By damaging the reputation of your employer, you're hurting yourself and countless other employees who come to work every day to do a good job. If you take issue with something going on at work, speak with the appropriate person and communicate your concerns in a professional manner.

- Don't make negative remarks about your company or its employees in public.
- Use **discretion** (being careful about what one says and does).
- Give your employer and your coworkers the benefit of the doubt; assume that everyone is there to do his or her best.
- If you have serious doubts about your employer and the way your company does business, it's probably best to look for employment at another company.

Evaluating Your Performance

Now that you're familiar with what it takes to demonstrate a strong work ethic, let's examine how health care employers evaluate job performance. If you take your job seriously and apply everything you are learning in this book, you should have no problem when it comes time for your performance evaluation. If you lack the competence or the commitment required to perform your job effectively, your deficiencies will soon become apparent.

The process used to conduct **performance evaluations** (measurements of success in executing job duties) varies from company to company. Sometimes it's called a *performance appraisal* or *performance management*. The purpose of a performance evaluation is not to determine how well an employee "is liked" or how his or her supervisor "feels" about the employee because this would involve **subjective** criteria (affected by a state of mind or feelings). Instead, employers evaluate job performance using **objective** criteria (what is real or actual; not affected by feelings), which is based on factors such as competence, behaviors (customer service, teamwork, problem solving), and traits (attitude, appearance, initiative). Evaluating competence and behaviors using objective criteria is fairly straightforward but assessing traits such as "appearance" and "attitude" without becoming subjective can be difficult.

It's not unusual for new employees to undergo a **probationary period** (a testing or trial period to meet requirements) whereby their attendance and performance are closely monitored for the first few months to make sure they are a good fit for the organization and the position. New employees are evaluated at the end of their probationary period and the decision is made to retain the employees or not. Having successfully completed their probationary period, employees are then subject to regular performance evaluations from that point forward, typically done on an annual basis.

Small organizations may evaluate performance on an informal basis. The supervisor observes the employee's performance over a period of time and provides verbal feedback regarding strengths, weaknesses, and areas for improvement. Informal evaluations may or may not be documented in writing and kept in the employee's personnel file. Larger companies typically evaluate performance on a more formal basis. The supervisor observes the employee's performance during the year, completes a written performance evaluation form, and meets with the employee to discuss the results. The performance evaluation form and notes from the meeting are documented in writing and kept in the employee's personnel file. Some companies give their employees the opportunity to do a self-evaluation. This can be very helpful in preparing for your evaluation meeting with your supervisor. Think about your performance over the past year and what you have accomplished. Jot down notes and bring them with you to the meeting.

RECENT DEVELOPMENTS

360-DEGREE FEEDBACK

Employers are now using **360-degree feedback** tools (feedback about an employee's job performance that is provided by **peers** [people at the same rank], subordinates, team members, customers, and others who have worked with the employee who is undergoing evaluation) as part of performance evaluations. People who have worked with the employee during the past year are asked to provide input to the employee's evaluation. Getting feedback from people in addition to the employee's supervisor helps reduce subjectivity and provides a broader view of the employee's performance. When employees work on teams, getting performance feedback from other team members helps evaluate the employee's team skills as well as his or her individual performance.

In addition to focusing on previous performance, the evaluation process also lays out plans for the coming year. Through discussions with supervisors, employees develop **goals** (aims, objects, or ends that one strives to attain) for the coming year to help them progress from where they are to where they eventually want to be. The goal-setting process helps employees overcome deficiencies, enhance skills, and work toward job promotions and career advancement.

Each company has its own rating scale. Typically, a few employees will receive an "outstanding" evaluation, most will receive an "average" evaluation, and a few may receive a "poor" evaluation. Performance evaluations may result in more than just feedback about how well you're doing on the job. Many companies now tie the amount of an individual's pay increase to the score on his or her performance evaluation. This is called performance-based pay, merit-based pay, or pay for performance. Employees who receive high scores on their performance evaluations receive higher pay raises than employees who receive lower scores. Employees with poor scores may not

CASE STUDY

It's been just over a year since Carla decided to stick with her job and she's glad she did. Joining a network turned out to be a positive change for everyone including the employees, doctors, and patients. Switching to electronic medical records was quite a challenge but the benefits are now obvious. Although Carla was nervous about having to learn some new computer skills, she sailed through the training and even helped her coworkers and the doctors complete theirs. With renewed confidence in her ability to learn new things, Carla is seriously considering enrolling in a bachelor's degree program at a local university using the tuition assistance benefit she gained when her employer joined the network.

Now it's time for Carla to undergo her first performance evaluation. She hasn't been late or missed a day of work since she started. She has a positive attitude, submits suggestions for improvement, and always speaks highly of her employer in public. She complies with policies and rules, accepts responsibility, and holds herself personally accountable for the quality of her work. The doctors and her manager have made lots of positive comments about her performance but Carla realizes she's in the early stages of her career and still has more to learn.

What can Carla do to prepare for her first performance evaluation? How can she find out what criteria will be used and how her performance will be scored? What materials could she gather to demonstrate the quality of her work and the impact she has made during the year? Should she mention that she joined a professional association and attended continuing education seminars every quarter? Should she bring up the fact that she's thinking about returning to school to work on an advanced degree? What would you do to prepare for your performance evaluation if you were in Carla's place?

receive a pay raise at all. When pay is tied to performance, it's even more important to focus on objective criteria rather than subjective criteria in the evaluation process.

Which behaviors result in outstanding evaluations? Keep reading this book because most everything you need to know to earn an outstanding evaluation is covered in these chapters. As you read, start evaluating your own strengths and weaknesses. Think about what you need to improve on and what steps you will take to do so.

When your performance review gets close, take the following steps to prepare:

- Review your job description and make sure you're familiar with the essential functions of your position.
- If your company uses a performance evaluation form, ask for a copy. Make sure you understand the performance criteria and how performance is evaluated and scored.

- If your company's performance evaluation process is computerized, make sure you have the computer skills you need to complete your part of the process.
- Complete your self-evaluation and make a copy for your supervisor.
- Think about the goals you set for the past year. Did you accomplish them? Why or why not? Jot down your accomplishments and note what you would like to achieve in the coming year.
- Keep a list of questions you might want to ask your supervisor when you meet.

The night before your review, get plenty of sleep and try to relax. This is when being prepared really helps. During the meeting with your supervisor keep these points in mind:

- Practice good listening skills, pay attention to everything your supervisor says, take notes, and ask for clarification when you don't understand something.
- If you disagree with something, state your reasons in an objective, respectful manner and avoid becoming defensive.
- Brace yourself for some negative feedback. If you've done your best all year long, you should also hear lots of positives.
- Accept **constructive criticism** (viewing one's weaknesses in a way that leads to positive improvement) and learn from it.
- Compare the score on your self-evaluation with the score your supervisor gave you and discuss any differences.
- If you disagree with what's been said during your evaluation, state your opinions clearly and objectively but don't expect your score to change.
- If you're expected to make improvements during the coming year, make sure you know exactly what's expected of you and how improvements will be measured.
- At the end of the session, summarize important next steps and thank your supervisor for the time he or she spent with you.

Keep in mind that some supervisors are more skilled and experienced than others in providing constructive feedback and coaching their subordinates for improvement. Performance evaluations can create some uncomfortable conflict. Employees aren't the only people who experience anxiety over these sessions—many supervisors do, too.

Remember, no one is perfect and everyone has more to learn. Even if your company doesn't have a performance evaluation process, you can (and should) request periodic feedback. This can be as simple as asking, "How do you think I'm doing?" You don't have to wait until your annual review time to ask. Solicit feedback from your supervisor and coworkers on a regular basis and then act on what they've told you. If your performance becomes an issue, chances are your supervisor will let you know as soon as the problem becomes apparent, but don't subscribe to the "no news is good news" theory. Soliciting feedback from those most familiar with your performance is the best way to increase your value to the organization.

Understanding the elements of a strong work ethic and performing well on the job are vital in developing your reputation as a health care professional. The next step is examining your personal traits and how they affect your work.

For More Information

Health Care Compliance Association
www.hcca-info.org
888-580-8373

HIPAA

U.S. Department of Health and Human Services
www.hhs.gov/ocr/privacy/hipaa/
understanding/index.html
877-696-6775

Sexual Harassment

U.S. Equal Employment Opportunity Commission
www.eeoc.gov/laws/types/sexual_
harassment.cfm
800-669-4000

REALITY CHECK

Perhaps you've already had one or more jobs where you've been held to certain performance standards and had to comply with company policies and procedures. If you appeared for work every day and on time, demonstrated competence and a commitment to your job, and proved to be a reliable and enthusiastic employee, then you probably earned a satisfactory performance evaluation and maybe a pay raise or job promotion. If so, this experience and what you learned from it will serve you well as you assume your new role in health care.

But as mentioned previously, working in health care presents some unique challenges. More than likely, you'll be working in a complex, stressful environment where everything that you say and do will make an impact on other people. It's like throwing a pebble in a pond and watching the ripple effect. You can see some of the ripples created because they happen right in front of you but other ripples are off in the distance, too far away to observe.

Your attitude and behaviors at work also cause ripples. When you smile and project a friendly attitude, for example, you create positive ripples. Conversely, when you complain and spread negativity, you create negative ripples. When you "go beyond the call of duty" to do something special for a patient or a coworker, you create positive ripples. When you get lazy and develop an "I don't care" attitude about your work, you create negative ripples. Like tossing a pebble in the pond, you won't always be able to observe much of the impact you've made, whether positive or negative. It all comes back to being intentional about everything you say and do. Stop and think before you act because the ripples *you* create should only be the positive ones.

Key Points

- Commit to your job and make it a high priority in your life.
- From a systems perspective, know where your role fits in.
- Be present in the moment.
- Stop and think before you act; everything you say and do should be intentional.
- Develop effective critical thinking skills to help solve problems.
- Report for work when scheduled and arrive on time.
- Adopt an optimistic attitude and display enthusiasm at work.
- Maintain your competency and always work within your scope of practice.
- Pay attention to quality and submit suggestions to improve it.
- Comply with all policies, laws, and rules that apply to your job.
- Avoid illegal, unethical, and inappropriate behavior.
- Represent your employer in a professional manner.
- Ask for feedback about your job performance and make improvements as needed.

Learning Activities

Using information from Chapter Two:
- Answer the Chapter Review Questions.
- Respond to the What If? Scenarios.
- Complete Chapter Two activities on the website.

Chapter Review Questions

Using information presented in Chapter Two, answer each of the following questions:

1. Define *interdependence* and *systems perspective* and explain their importance in health care.

2. Explain why it's important to be "present in the moment" at work.

3. Define *critical thinking* and list three things that critical thinkers do to make good decisions.

4. List five factors that demonstrate a strong work ethic.

5. Describe the attitudinal differences between optimists and pessimists.

6. Discuss the importance of confidentiality and HIPAA.

7. Identify how competence and scope of practice impact quality of care.

8. List two things you should do when representing your employer.

9. Explain the purpose of performance evaluations and list three ways to prepare for one.

10. Differentiate between objective and subjective evaluation criteria.

What If? Scenarios

Think about what you would do in the following situations and record your answers.

1. You were out with friends until very late last night and had to report for work this morning at 7:00 AM. You know your coworkers won't arrive for another half an hour. You've got just enough time for a quick run to the corner coffee shop before your coworkers arrive.

2. You promised your coworkers you'd work the day shift on Thanksgiving so they could be home with their families. Then two days before the holiday, an old friend from out of town calls to say he'd like you to be his guest for lunch on Thanksgiving Day.

3. Your shift ends in 30 minutes and you've got about 30 minutes of work left to do but you haven't gotten to take your afternoon break yet.

4. Your niece needs to sell 10 more packs of popcorn to earn a fund-raising prize at school. You're pretty sure your coworkers would buy some.

5. Your supervisor has asked you out on a date twice. Both times you declined saying you'd prefer to not date people from work. Now he's asking again and reminds you that your performance review is coming up next month.

6. The office manager tells you to enter a code on an insurance form that she knows is not correct. If you enter the incorrect code as she has told you to do, the clinic will receive more money from the insurance company than it would if you enter the correct code.

7. One of your neighbors is admitted to the unit where you work. A relative of yours calls to tell you he's heard a rumor that the neighbor has a communicable disease. Because you work on the unit and have access to records, your relative asks you to find out if the rumor is true.

8. A new piece of equipment has been installed in your department and you missed the in-service when your coworkers were trained to operate it. The next day there's a procedure to be done using this equipment and it's your responsibility to do it.

9. A coworker invites you to a party. When you arrive, you notice three people that you work with complaining about low wages and telling a group of strangers that one of the surgeons at your hospital made a mistake last week and lied to the patient's family to cover it up.

10. A doctor mistakes you for a registered nurse and tells you to prepare a medication for him to administer to a patient. Even though you prepared medications in your previous job, it's not within the scope of practice for your current job.

PEARSON
myhealthprofessionskit™

Go to www.myhealthprofessionskit.com to access the Companion Website created for this textbook. Simply select "Basic Health Science" from the choice of disciplines. Find this book and log in using your username and password to access video scenarios, self-assessment quizzes, and more.

Personal Traits of the Health Care Professional

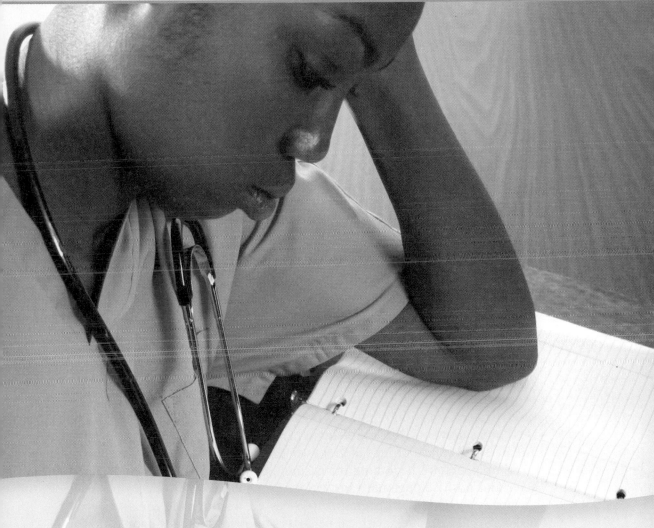

"The ultimate measure of a man is not where he stands in moments of comfort and convenience, but where he stands at times of challenge and controversy."

Martin Luther King Jr.,
Civil rights leader, 1929–1968

CHAPTER OBJECTIVES

Having completed this chapter, you will be able to:

- Define *character* and *personal values* and explain how these affect your reputation as a professional.
- List four examples of lack of character in the workplace.
- Explain how your character traits and personal values affect your behavior and attitude.

- List three important questions to ask yourself when making difficult ethical decisions.
- Give three examples of dishonest behaviors and describe the impact of dishonesty in the workplace.
- Define *ethics* and *morals* and discuss how they impact judgment and behavior.
- Define *fraud* and give three examples.
- List three examples of complex ethical, moral, and legal dilemmas in health care.

KEY TERMS

character	ethics	loyalty	priorities
cheating	integrity	morals	trustworthiness
conscience	judgment	personal values	

Character and Personal Values

Professionalism brings together who you are as a person and how you contribute those traits in the workplace. Before you can achieve success "doing" something, you have to "be" something, and being a health care professional depends greatly on who you are as a person. It takes a long time to develop a good reputation and only a split second to lose it. Much of this comes down to your **character** (a person's moral behavior and qualities) and **personal values** (things of great worth and importance).

Employers are becoming increasingly concerned about a lack of character and positive personal values in the workplace. Each year in businesses throughout the United States, employees are responsible for a variety of dishonest, illegal, and unethical behaviors and this includes people working for health care companies. Here are just a few examples:

- Hidden video cameras in hospitals reveal employees stealing computers, office supplies, syringes, medications, and patients' personal possessions.
- Job applicants falsify information on employment applications and overstate their education and work records.
- Countless numbers of fraudulent worker compensation claims are filed each year.
- Employees bring weapons to work and arguments, fistfights, workplace violence, and sexual harassment are becoming more commonplace.

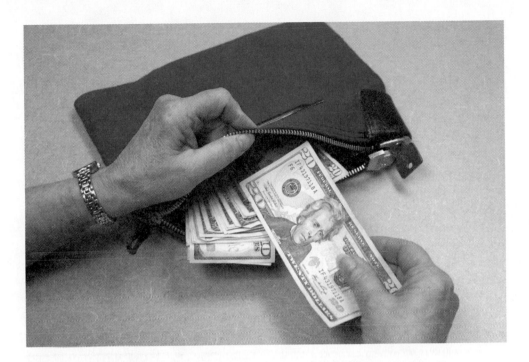

Figure 3-1 ■ Preparing cash for deposit

Increasingly health care employers are running criminal history background checks, credit checks, and drug screens on job candidates before they start work. Employers are also placing more emphasis on the character of their employees to help reduce theft, absenteeism, dishonesty, workplace violence, substance abuse, safety infractions, negligence, and low productivity. More and more, employers are hiring for character, praising for character, and promoting for character. Character reflects a person's **morals** (capability of differentiating between right and wrong) and influences their **integrity** (of sound moral principle) and **trustworthiness** (ability to have confidence in the honesty, integrity, and reliability of another person), two key factors in professionalism.

How do character, personal values, reputation, morals, integrity, and trustworthiness apply to you as a person? How do they affect the way you approach your work? Do you know the difference between right and wrong? Are you honest? Can you be trusted? If you make a bad decision, can you overcome it and get back on track?

Character Traits

Character traits lead to a person's behavior, thoughts, and emotions. Here are a couple of examples:

- "Amiable" (good humored and friendly) versus "ill-natured" (unpleasant disposition)

Would you like to work with an amiable person, one who is good humored, friendly, and able to establish positive relationships with patients and coworkers? Or would you rather work with a grumpy person who doesn't seem to like being around other people?

- "Ambitious" (strong desire to achieve) versus "shiftless" (lacking ambition and initiative)

Would you prefer to have an ambitious coworker, one who strives to exceed expectations? Or would you prefer a shiftless coworker who fails to take initiative and doesn't seem to care?

If you were choosing a new team member, which of these character traits would you look for?

You can find lengthy lists of character traits. Box 3-1 shows several examples that identify positive and negative aspects of each type of trait. Think about each trait. Which of these describe you? How might each trait affect customer service, relationships, and morale in the workplace?

Box 3-1 ■ Character Traits

Appreciative/Ungrateful
- Feeling or expressing gratitude
- Not thankful or appreciative

Caring/Callous
- Feeling concern and interest
- Insensitive and emotionally hardened

Cheerful/Grumpy
- In good spirits
- Ill-tempered

Conscientious/Careless
- Taking extreme care and attention to details
- Lack of attention and forethought

Courteous/Impolite
- Polite, uses good manners
- Failure to demonstrate good manners

Dependable/Undependable
- Worthy of trust, can be counted on
- Not worthy of reliance or trust

Diligent/Neglectful
- Careful in one's work
- Failure to show care or attention

Generous/Selfish
- Willing to give and share with others
- Concerned with one's self to the detriment of others

Honest/Deceitful
- Marked by truth
- Deliberately false and fraudulent

Humble/Boastful
- Marked by modesty and a lack of arrogance
- Exhibiting self-importance

Impartial/Biased
- Free from favoritism and preconceived opinions
- Favoring one person or side over the other

Integrity/Immoral
- Of sound moral principle
- Failure to differentiate between right and wrong

Loyal/Disloyal
- Faithful to people whom one is under obligation to defend or support
- Deserting people whom one is under obligation to defend or support

Reliable/Unreliable
- Can be counted on, trustworthy
- Not worthy of reliance or trust

Respectful/Disrespectful
- Feeling or showing honor or esteem
- Failure to feel or show respect, rude and discourteous

Sincere/Hypocritical
- Open and genuine, not deceitful
- Pretending to be or feel something that is not real

Self-disciplined/Indulgent
- Ability to control one's impulses, avoids temptations
- Inability to control one's impulses, gives in to temptations

(Continued)

Box 3-1 ■ *(Continued)*

Tolerant/Intolerant
- Showing respect for the rights, opinions, and practices of others
- Narrow-minded, unwilling to show respect for the rights, opinions, and practices of others

Truthful/Untruthful
- Conforming to the truth, does not lie
- Intentionally lies and spreads false information

Reputation

No single factor is more important in being recognized as a professional than your reputation. After years of being an honest, law-abiding individual, all it takes is one dishonest act or a single incident of unprofessional behavior to shake people's confidence in you and lose their trust. This is why professionals must work hard each and every day to do what's right and to maintain the trust and respect of others.

If you've developed a pattern of behavior over the years of lying, **cheating** (deceiving by trickery), stealing, and taking advantage of other people, then changing your character at this point in your life is going to be quite a challenge, but it's possible. Our sense of acceptable behavior starts at a very young age when our parents and other influential people teach us the difference between right and wrong. As children, we experiment with different kinds of behavior to see what reactions we get. If those who raise us believe in discipline, we soon learn the consequences of "doing something bad." We are taught to get along with other children, share our toys, wash our hands before we eat, and make our beds. Unacceptable behavior results in "getting grounded" and losing privileges such as playing with friends or watching television.

Over the years, we learn to make **judgment** calls to compare our options and decide which is best. We learn the concept of self-control and the importance of avoiding temptation. Through relationships with other people, we learn about fairness, respect, **ethics** (standards of conduct and moral judgment), and **loyalty** (showing faith to people that one is under obligation to defend or support). We learn to care, to give, and to appreciate. And before long, our character, values, and **priorities** (having precedence in time, order, and importance) begin to define who we are as people and how we conduct our lives.

Judgment

As adults, we're faced with multiple decisions every day—what to do, why or why not to do it, how to do it, when to do it, where to do it, with whom to do it, and so on. Some of the decisions we have to make are small ones, but other decisions, especially those involving relationships with other people, require more thought and carry significant consequences—how to resolve a disagreement, when to say "no," and when to ask for help.

Several questions need to be considered when using judgment to make decisions:

- What are my choices?
- How do the options compare with one another?
- What might happen?
- Who might be affected?
- How would it make me feel?
- How would my decision be viewed by other people?

When the decisions you face involve your job, more questions arise:

- What would my supervisor think?
- How would my coworkers feel?
- How would this affect our patients?
- Could I lose my job?

Conscience

Most people have a **conscience** (moral judgment that prohibits or opposes the violation of a previously recognized ethical principle)—a little voice that gnaws away at you, keeps you from sleeping at night, and constantly says, "You *know* this *isn't* the right thing to do!" Your conscience can be quite reliable in reminding you of the difference between right and wrong. When you're facing some really difficult situations, more questions need to be answered:

- How would this look if it appeared in the newspaper?
- How would my children feel?
- Would my family support me?
- Could I look myself in the mirror?
- Would I be able to sleep at night?

The problem is that some people either have no conscience or have learned to ignore their conscience. It starts with something minor, such as telling a little lie or stealing something small. And then it grows and grows until it becomes a way of life. Eventually dishonest and unethical behavior will become obvious, but in the meantime countless people could be affected.

The good news is that the majority of Americans are honest, law-abiding people with good character and sound moral values. People who sincerely want to do what's right in their lives:

- Face temptations but summon up the courage to say "no!"
- Avoid engaging in dishonest behavior just because "everyone else does."

- Forgive others and move on without harboring anger and resentment.
- Look out for themselves but treat other people with fairness and respect.
- Exercise good judgment and make the right decisions for the right reasons.

In the health care workplace, personal traits such as character, values, morals, ethics, integrity, and trustworthiness are absolutely vital. If you were sick or injured, what kind of people would you want caring for you? If you owned a health care business, what kind of people would you want working for you?

CONSIDER THIS

MEDICARE FRAUD

Massive, nationwide arrests of doctors, nurses, physical therapists, and other health care providers for Medicare fraud are on the rise. Medicare fraud is estimated to cause an additional $60 to $90 billion per year in unnecessary government health care costs. Here are some examples:

- A proctologist earned $6.5 million for hemorrhoid removals, most of which never occurred.
- A podiatrist collected $700,000 for partial toenail removals, which were actually toenail clippings.
- Physical therapists collected $57 million for little more than back rubs.
- Doctors and nurses from a home health care agency collected $25 million by writing fake prescriptions for expensive treatments for homebound patients.

The federal government is stepping up efforts to uncover and stop these kinds of fraudulent practices.

Trust

Part of developing a professional reputation is convincing people that they can trust you and the quality of the decisions you make. In today's society, many people have become increasingly suspicious of other people, warning, "Don't trust anyone!" Unfortunately, that perspective gets reinforced each time we set ourselves up to believe in someone or depend on someone, only to end up disappointed or let down. It's important to be reliable and to follow through when someone is counting on you. When your word is "as good as gold," your supervisor and coworkers know they can trust you to keep your promises and meet your obligations.

- If you promise to give a coworker a ride to work, don't forget to pick him up.
- If you receive training on a new procedure and your supervisor trusts you to perform it properly, make sure you apply what you learned.

- If you tell a patient you'll relay a message to her nurse, follow through.

If you want people to view you as a professional, make sure you can be trusted.

Honesty

Earning respect relies greatly on being viewed as an honest person. As mentioned previously, dishonesty has become a problem in the health care workplace. The cost of health care is high enough without employers having to pay for extra supplies, food, and equipment stolen by their employees. Most health care workers would deny that they steal from their employers or patients but theft goes well beyond stealing a computer or a patient's wallet. Here are some examples of theft that you might not think of:

- Manipulating your time card to get paid for more hours than you worked
- Sleeping on the job, taking unauthorized breaks, or leaving your work area without permission
- Taking food off a dietary cart delivered for a lunch meeting
- Taking supplies off a patient's bedside table to use at home

Anytime you take *anything* that doesn't belong to you without proper authorization, it can be construed as theft. Is a free sandwich or box of cotton swabs worth losing your job over? What about an extra hour of pay that you didn't really deserve? This is when honesty and good judgment enter the picture. Even if taking something that doesn't belong to you appears harmless, what might be the consequences?

RECENT DEVELOPMENTS

EMBEZZLEMENT

According to a recent study, as many as 80% of group practice physicians could be victimized by embezzlers during their careers, mostly involving receptionists and office managers who handle cash before and after office hours. The problem is sometimes detected when office personnel refuse to take vacation or sick time because they fear their dishonest acts will be discovered when they're away from the office. To reduce the potential for theft, physicians may run periodic credit checks on employees who handle cash and they rotate assignments so that more than one person is responsible for overseeing the finances.

When employees spend time on the clock doing something other than assigned job duties, they aren't just wasting time, they're stealing from their company by collecting pay for nonproductive time. Examples include texting friends, visiting social networking sites, accessing pornographic websites, gambling, shopping online, and using company computers for other inappropriate activities. Employees may also be caught sleeping, watching television, and engaging in sexual activity while on the job.

Lying and cheating are two more dishonest behaviors that can get you in big trouble. Little, seemingly harmless "white lies" usually snowball into big, complicated lies that can become difficult to manage. Lies are eventually uncovered and, before long, people will wonder if they can believe *anything* you say. Being truthful is always the best approach.

Cheating is an example of dishonest behavior that results from giving in to temptation. Maybe you have to pass a written test to prove your competency for a job promotion but didn't have time to prepare. Dozens of people will be taking the test at the same time and no one would notice if you sneaked some notes into the room with you. After all, you could actually learn the material later on, after passing the test. If your supervisor finds out that you've cheated on the test, you'll be in big trouble. Forget the job promotion because your main concern will be keeping the job you've got. If you think your coworkers who are competing for the same job promotion will stand by quietly and let you get away with cheating on the test, think again. They prepared for the test and you didn't. If you get the job promotion as a

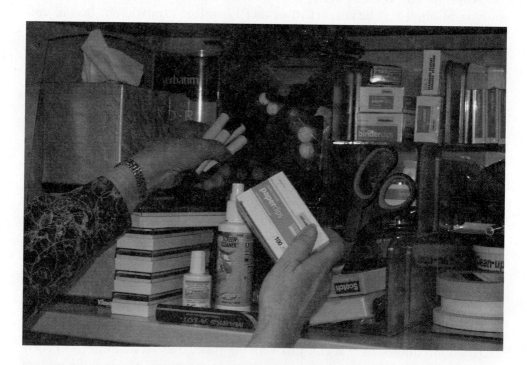

Figure 3-2 ■ Taking supplies from work to use at home

CASE STUDY

It's been almost four months since Carla underwent her first annual performance review. Positive feedback from the doctors and her office manager and coworkers resulted in an outstanding evaluation. Carla received the highest score that the practice has ever given to a new medical assistant with just one year of experience. She received a modest pay raise and spent part of her next paycheck on the textbook that's required for the college course she just enrolled in.

Things were going really well until last week when Carla overheard one of the network's purchasing agents on the telephone with a salesperson from a local computer company. Carla heard the purchasing agent tell the salesperson that she would buy 100 computers for the network if the salesperson would agree to give her husband the same quantity discount for the five new computers he needs for their family-owned grocery.

At first, Carla didn't pay much attention but the more she thought about it, she realized that what the purchasing agent was doing wasn't right. She was using her authority as her company's purchasing agent for her own personal gain and that seemed like a conflict of interest to Carla. Now she can't decide what she should do, if anything. She's still relatively new, really likes her job, and doesn't want to cause trouble but she can't help but wonder what other dishonest acts the purchasing agent might be involved in. If someone finds out that she suspected the purchasing agent of unethical behavior but didn't report it, Carla's afraid that she might get in trouble, too.

What, if anything, should Carla do? Should she mind her own business and remain quiet? Or should she report the matter to a superior, confront the purchasing agent about the conflict of interest, or take some other action? What would you do if you were in Carla's place?

result of cheating, your lack of competence may quickly become obvious and other people may suffer. Your professional reputation will be seriously damaged, perhaps beyond repair. Can you cheat just a little and get away with it? Ask your conscience.

A serious example of dishonest behavior is falsifying information, also known as *fraud*. Fraud is not only dishonest, it's illegal. A few examples of fraud include:

- Misrepresenting your education, credentials, or work experience on a job application, résumé, or other document
- Billing an insurance company for a patient procedure that never occurred
- Back-dating a legal document, entering incorrect data on equipment maintenance records, or changing the results of a research study

As with stealing and cheating, there may be more to fraud than you realize. Fraud includes:

- Signing someone else's name without his or her permission
- Turning in a time card that you know is inaccurate
- Telling your supervisor that you passed a competency assessment when you really didn't

Since fraud is illegal, a fraud conviction can not only cost you your job, it can also cost you your freedom.

Ethics

Another personal trait that factors into your reputation as a professional is ethics—standards of conduct and moral judgment. Would you do the following?

- Inform the cafeteria cashier that she gave you too much change
- Look in a confidential file that lists your supervisor's salary
- Clock out for a friend who wants to leave work early

THINK ABOUT IT

THE RIGHT THING TO DO

Do you always follow the rules? Or do you "bend" them when you're sure you won't get caught? For example, do you:

- Exceed the speed limit in construction zones when no police are present?
- Park in a handicapped spot when no one is looking?
- Borrow someone else's ID to get his or her discount on your purchase?
- Return a mail-order item that your child broke, claiming it was damaged in shipment?

Professionals don't do the right thing because they're afraid of getting caught. They do the right thing because *it's the right thing to do.*

If it seems as if unethical behaviors overlap with lying, cheating, stealing, and other dishonest acts discussed earlier in this chapter, your observations are correct. It's hard to separate one type of unprofessional behavior from another. Consider the following:

- Failing to return extra change in the cafeteria isn't just unethical, it's theft.
- Looking in a confidential file isn't just unethical, it's a breach of confidentiality.
- Clocking out for a friend isn't just unethical, it's fraud.

The point is that every decision you make and every action you take can have a huge effect. One bad judgment call can erode someone's trust in you.

One unethical decision can destroy your reputation. One illegal act can cause you to be fired from your job—or worse.

If you find yourself in a difficult situation weighing one option against another, and you're not quite sure which course of action to pursue, consider the following questions:

- Is it honest?
- Is it ethical?
- Does it reflect good character?
- Is it based on sound moral values?
- How would it affect my reputation?
- Would it damage the trust others have in me?
- What impact would my actions have on others?
- Would I be respected for my decision?
- What does my conscience tell me to do?
- What would a professional do?

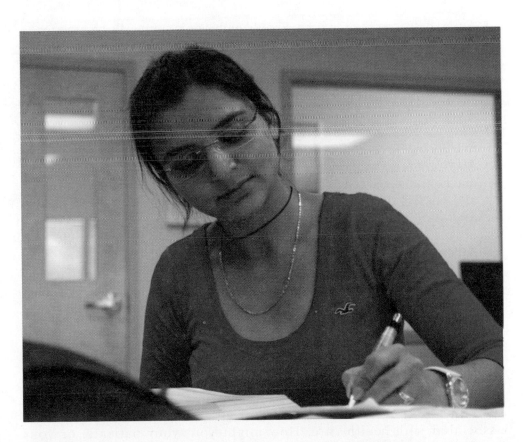

Figure 3-3 ■ Weighing options to make the best decision.

Ethical, Moral, and Legal Dilemmas

Most of the information presented so far in this chapter relates to who you are as a person and how your character traits and values affect your work and your reputation as a professional. But people who work in the health care industry, as well as other stakeholders, also face a multitude of complex ethical, moral, and legal dilemmas that stretch well beyond how just one person thinks or behaves. Depending on the profession you have chosen, you may become directly involved in some issues yourself. Here are some examples of the difficult and controversial questions that people are grappling with:

- *Abortion:* Should abortion remain legal? Should an abortion to save the mother's life or in cases of rape be legal? Should late-term abortions be legal? Should tax dollars be used to pay for abortions?
- *Genetic testing:* Should insurance companies be permitted to cancel a patient's coverage due to the results of genetic testing? When prenatal genetic testing uncovers serious medical problems, should the fetus be aborted?
- *Embryonic stem cell research:* Should embryonic stem cells be used for medical research considering that the embryos must be destroyed as part of the process?
- *Rationing:* Should health care be rationed to reduce costs and reserve limited resources for those patients who would benefit the most?
- *Cloning:* Should scientists clone human beings to produce organs for use in transplants and other medical procedures?
- *Medical marijuana:* Should patients who could benefit from using marijuana to reduce pain and increase appetite be permitted to buy and possess the drug even though marijuana is illegal?
- *End-of-life care:* Should life-sustaining treatments such as feeding tubes or ventilators be withdrawn to facilitate the death of terminally ill patients?
- *Euthanasia:* Is assisting someone with suicide ever justifiable and, if so, under what conditions?
- *Organ transplants:* When several patients are awaiting an organ for transplantation, which patients should get priority? Should an alcoholic patient about to die from liver disease be eligible for a transplant?
- *Refusing treatment:* Should parents be allowed to refuse treatment for a sick child based on their religious beliefs?

These are just a few of the complex ethical, moral, and legal issues associated with health care. How might you, your patients, or your employer become directly involved in some of these controversial issues?

Based on your own personal values, morals, and ethics, how would you answer these questions? What would you say to someone whose opinions are different from yours? Is it possible to decide who is right and who is wrong?

Having taken a closer look at your personal traits and how they affect your behavior, attitudes, and opinions, let's move on to examine what it takes to form and maintain effective interpersonal relationships at work.

For More Information

Medical Ethics
The American Academy of Medical Ethics
www.ethicalhealthcare.org
423-844-1095

Medicare Fraud and Abuse
U.S. Department of Health and Human Services and the U.S. Department of Justice
www.StopMedicareFraud.gov

Office of the Inspector General
800-447-8477
http://www.oig.hhs.gov/

REALITY CHECK

This chapter could provide a lot more examples of how your character and personal values affect who you are as a person and how you perform at work. But you already know what kind of person you are and you know the difference between right and wrong. You also know what's expected of health care professionals when it comes to ethics, honesty, and morals. You can either choose to live up to those high standards or you can try to slide by with less. No one can make that decision for you. If you've made some poor decisions in the past and failed to live up to professional standards, it's time to make some changes and get your life back on track.

Key Points

- Keep in mind that it takes time to develop a professional reputation but only a split second to lose it.
- Review the list of positive character traits and decide which ones you need to improve upon.
- Use good judgment in making decisions.
- Listen to your conscience and avoid temptations to do the wrong thing.
- Make sure that your word is "as good as gold" and follow through on your commitments.
- Don't take anything that doesn't belong to you without proper authorization.
- Don't lie, cheat, steal, commit fraud, or engage in any other illegal or unethical acts.
- Be aware of the ethical, moral, and legal dilemmas that might affect your patients, your employer, and your work.

Learning Activities

Using information from Chapter Three:
- Answer the Chapter Review Questions.
- Respond to the What If? Scenarios.
- Complete Chapter Three activities on the website.

Chapter Review Questions

Using information presented in Chapter Three, answer each of the following questions:

1. Define *character* and *personal values* and explain how these affect your reputation as a professional.

2. List four examples of lack of character in the workplace.

3. Explain how your character traits and personal values affect your behavior and attitude.

4. List three important questions to ask yourself when making difficult ethical decisions.

5. Give three examples of dishonest behaviors and describe the impact of dishonesty in the workplace.

6. Define *ethics* and *morals* and discuss how they impact judgment and behavior.

7. Define *fraud* and give three examples.

8. List three examples of complex ethical, moral, and legal dilemmas in health care.

What If? Scenarios

Think about what you would do in the following situations and record your answers:

1. You witness a coworker taking money from the petty cash box in your department. She says she needs to borrow the money to get her car fixed and she'll pay it back when she gets her next paycheck. She reminds you that she did you a big favor when you first started your job and asks that you not report her to the supervisor.

2. You need to have your time card signed by the end of the day. You know your supervisor would sign it, but she's tied up in a meeting and your shift ends in 10 minutes.

3. You have one more paper to turn in for a course you're taking that's required for your job. You keep the weekend open to write it but a dear friend calls and says he'll be in town for the weekend and would like to spend it with you. You have a copy of a paper that someone else wrote for the same course two years ago that earned a grade of "B." The instructor is new and would never know that you didn't write the paper yourself.

4. Your supervisor asked you to attend a meeting in her place but you forgot to go. You know she'll be upset with you because she needs the information that was handed out. When you see her she asks, "So what did you think of the meeting?"

5. A patient on your unit gets discharged. While cleaning the room for the next patient, you find an expensive watch in the drawer in the bedside table. It's a woman's watch and the former patient was a man.

6. When you open up your paycheck, you realize that you got paid for a day that you didn't work.

7. As a research assistant, your salary is funded by a federal grant. If the research gets positive results, the grant and your job will get renewed for another year. The research director tells you to change some of the data to indicate better results.

8. When it's time for your competency evaluation, your supervisor announces that you and your coworkers will be checking each other off. Your coworkers get together and decide just to give each other a satisfactory evaluation without actually checking each person's competency level.

9. Your sons are returning to school tomorrow after summer break. You haven't had time to shop for school supplies and are short on cash. Your company is overstocked with office supplies and no one would miss a few pencils, pens, and tablets of paper.

10. Your best friend, who works in the same department you do, asks you to clock her out at 3:00 PM so that she can leave work at 2:00 PM to attend her daughter's dance recital.

PEARSON
myhealthprofessionskit™

Go to www.myhealthprofessionskit.com to access the Companion Website created for this textbook. Simply select "Basic Health Science" from the choice of disciplines. Find this book and log in using your username and password to access video scenarios, self-assessment quizzes, and more.

Relationships, Teamwork, and Communication Skills

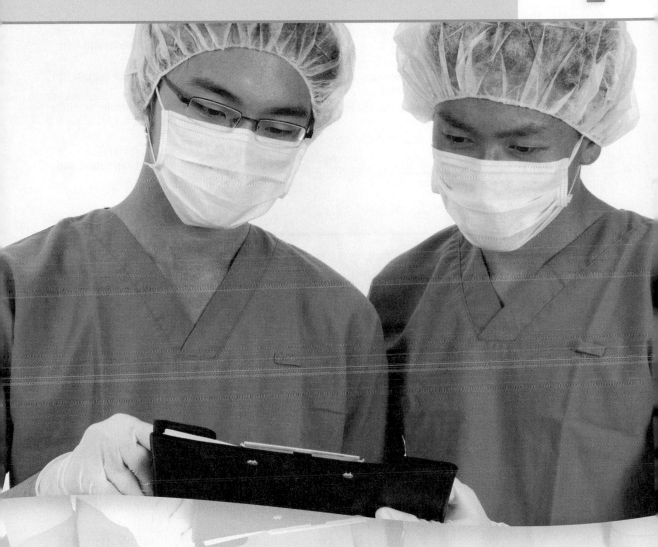

"Think enthusiastically about everything, but especially about your job. If you do so, you'll put a touch of glory in your life. If you love your job with enthusiasm, you'll shake it to pieces."

Normal Vincent Peale,
Clergyman and champion of positive thinking, 1898–1993

CHAPTER OBJECTIVES

Having completed this chapter, you will be able to:

- Discuss the concept of interdependence and list three ways to strengthen relationships at work.
- List two ways to demonstrate loyalty to your coworkers and two ways to demonstrate loyalty to your employer.
- Identify two types of workplace teams and give an example of each.
- Define the term *inclusive* and give two examples.
- Explain the role of courtesy, etiquette, and manners in the workplace.

- Define *consensus* and explain why it's important but difficult to achieve.
- List three problems that may occur when communicating electronically and describe three ways to prevent them from happening.
- Define *conflict resolution* and explain its importance.
- Name the four styles of communication and describe the potential impact of each style.
- Identify which communication style is most effective in conflict resolution and explain why.

KEY TERMS

body language	confrontation	etiquette	interpersonal relationships
civility	consensus	golden rule	manners
cliques	cooperation	group norms	polite
colleagues	courtesy	inclusive	synergy
conflict resolution	diversity		

Interpersonal Relationships

Now that we've examined character traits and how they're applied in the workplace, it's time to discuss how health care professionals work with other people. Your interactions with other people and the relationships you form with coworkers are the basis for success in the workplace. Interdependence is essential. No one person can do it all. Only groups of people working together can get the job done and done well.

Professionals devote a lot of energy to establishing positive **interpersonal relationships** (connections between or among people) and treating each other in a caring, respectful manner. Your ability to work well with coworkers contributes greatly to your reputation as a professional. Courtesy, etiquette, manners, cooperation, and loyalty are key factors in a professional work environment. Let's take a closer look at the need to work well with other people.

Coworkers as Customers

If you're employed on a full-time basis, you probably spend as much time with your coworkers as you do with your family and friends. People want to feel

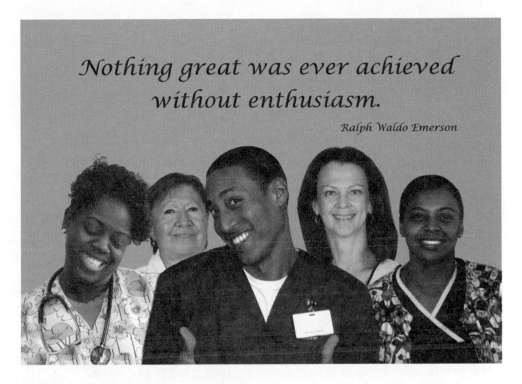

Nothing great was ever achieved without enthusiasm.

Ralph Waldo Emerson

Figure 4-1 ■ Enthusiastic attitudes create a positive work environment

good about coming to work, so it's important to create a positive, enjoyable work environment. Nothing can make your job more pleasant or miserable than your relationships with coworkers. Think about the relationships you've had in the past. Why did those relationships work well or not work well? Effective relationships are based on many of the factors already discussed in this text—trust, honesty, ethics, and morals—but several other traits and skills are also necessary.

You already know that patients, visitors, and guests are the customers of the health care company that you work for but have you realized that coworkers are your customers as well? That might seem strange but your coworkers are your "internal" customers and they deserve to be treated with the same respect and compassion that you would give your patients and other customers.

As mentioned earlier, your attitude at work is important. Displaying a friendly, positive attitude, saying hello to people you pass in the hallway, and smiling every chance you get goes a long way in creating a pleasant environment at work. Always look for the best in people, give them the benefit of the doubt, and assume that everyone is there to do his or her best.

Professionals need to be viewed as team players. It's best to cooperate with your coworkers and avoid whining, complaining, and questioning authority. Complainers "poison" the workplace and stir up discontent. If you get labeled as a complainer or troublemaker, your opportunities for advancement could be limited.

Inclusion and Friendliness

In order to form effective relationships with coworkers, it's best to be **inclusive**. Instead of excluding people and participating in **cliques** (small, exclusive circles of people), invite your coworkers to join you for lunch and make them feel welcome. Don't leave people out of the group. Excluding people can hurt their feelings and undermine their self-esteem. How you treat coworkers can have a direct impact on how they feel about themselves. If you want your coworkers to feel confident and good about themselves, then include them in your activities at work, reinforce their strengths and abilities, and help support their growth and advancement.

CONSIDER THIS

You and your coworkers don't need to be friends outside of work. Relationships with coworkers can enrich your professional life but friendship is not the goal of your relationships at work. In fact, you might not even like some of the people with whom you have to work but you need to find ways to get along with them and respect the knowledge, skills, and talents they bring to the workplace.

Because health care workers must depend on one another to get their work done, they must be willing to openly share information. Unfortunately, some people hoard information because it gives them a sense of power. They know something that you don't know and that makes them feel important, but this attitude is counterproductive to relationships and teamwork. It's also important to share space, equipment, and supplies. After all, you're all there for the same purpose—to serve patients and other customers, so there's no need for competition.

Laugh at yourself, be a good sport, and maintain your sense of humor. Avoid arrogance and don't be a snob. When you accomplish a goal, take pride but don't brag. Never look down on your coworkers or treat people in a demeaning way because they have less education, income, or status than you. There will always be people above and below you in the hierarchy of your organization and *every person* plays a critical role in accomplishing the company's mission. Remember the **golden rule:** treat other people the way you want to be treated. Better yet, treat people the way *they* want to be treated.

Building effective relationships doesn't happen overnight. It is hard work and you have to hang in there. Be patient and forgiving with yourself and your coworkers. No one is perfect—not even you! Get to know people better. You may discover a whole different side of someone's personality. Let your coworkers get to know you, too. The better your relationships, the more likely your coworkers will be there for you when you need them and vice versa.

Loyalty

Showing loyalty to the people who have helped you goes a long way in developing a professional reputation. One way to demonstrate loyalty to your coworkers is to be there for them when situations become stressful. Everyone who works in health care needs some encouragement and support from time to time. Getting the kind of emotional support that you need from people who don't work in health care themselves can be difficult. Even though family and friends may want to be helpful, it's hard to relate to the stress of working in health care unless you've experienced it yourself. This is especially true for employees who work on burn units and with critically ill children and patients facing death. Professionals need to be there for one another, to lend a helping hand or a shoulder to cry on. When someone you work with needs support, be ready to help. Most of time it means just listening and understanding.

The concept of loyalty also relates to your relationship with your employer. Remember the statement, "*You* are the company you work for"? Stop and think about it. You don't actually work for a company, you work for the *people* who own and manage the company. Companies are just legal entities that own assets such as buildings, property, and equipment. You don't work for a building, you work for people! Professionals are able to make that distinction and they feel a sense of loyalty to the people they *work for* as well as to the people they *work with*. You may not agree with management's policies, but don't forget that it's the people who manage your company who are providing you with a job and an opportunity to earn a living.

How can you demonstrate loyalty to your employer?

- Let management know you appreciate them and are proud to be part of the organization. Managers are people, too, and they appreciate being appreciated.
- Give management the benefit of the doubt. Until you've walked in their shoes, you can't fully appreciate the challenges they face every day.
- If your employer invests in your education and training, help pay back the investment by continuing to work there for a reasonable length of time. If a local competitor offers you extra pay to switch companies, remember who invested in your education and show your loyalty. Someday you may need a recommendation from your current employer. If management views you as a loyal employee, it can only help.
- Represent your employer in a professional manner. Always speak highly of management when in public and do your best to enhance your company's reputation.

Cooperation

Cooperation (acting or working together for a common purpose) is essential in maintaining effective relationships at work. Offer to help your coworkers even if they haven't asked for assistance. When you've got a tough job to do or you're running late, isn't it a welcome relief to hear someone say, "Need a hand?" Offer to rotate shifts and holiday coverage—your coworkers will appreciate the consideration. Make personal sacrifices, such as coming in early or staying late, to help a coworker—sensitivity and kindness are rewarded many times over. Learn to rely on one another, especially in emergencies and other stressful situations. Gain an appreciation for the strengths, abilities, and personal traits that each coworker contributes. Volunteer to serve on committees and sign up for employer-sponsored recreational activities to meet people and establish more relationships. Join people during your lunch break and widen your circle of **colleagues** (fellow workers in the same profession). You'll find there's **synergy** (people working together in a cooperative action) in working with other people. After all, a group can accomplish so much more than individuals working on their own.

THINK ABOUT IT

"ALL I REALLY NEED TO KNOW I LEARNED IN KINDERGARTEN"

In his 2003 book entitled, "All I Really Need to Know I Learned in Kindergarten", Robert Fulghum states, "All I really need to know I learned in kindergarten: Share everything. Play fair. Don't hit people. Put things back where you found them. Clean up your own mess. Don't take things that aren't yours. Say you're sorry when you hurt somebody. Wash your hands before you eat. Flush. Be aware of wonder. When you go out into the world, watch out for traffic, hold hands, and stick together." Much of this advice applies in today's health care workplace.

Etiquette and Manners

A growing number of Americans, especially employers, are expressing concerns about the erosion of **civility** in our society—the decline of courteous, **polite** (having good manners) behavior. This concern is especially problematic in health care where people must work together, often under stressful conditions, to meet customer needs. So employers are increasingly emphasizing the roles that **courtesy** (polite behavior, gestures, and remarks), **etiquette** (acceptable standards of behavior in a polite society), and **manners** (standards of behavior based on thoughtfulness and consideration of other people) play in the workplace

If it seems as if the definitions of courtesy, etiquette, and manners overlap with one another, that's okay. What's important is the role that polite behavior plays at work, at home, and in all aspects of your life. Consider the following examples.

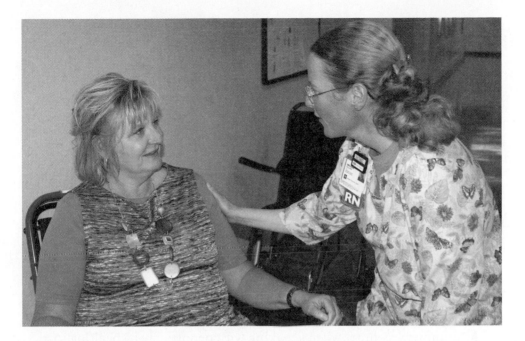

Figure 4-2 ■ Nurse showing care and concern

COURTESY

- Ask others before changing the room temperature, adjusting window blinds, turning on the TV, or playing music.
- Respect other people's possessions; return borrowed items quickly and if you break something, repair it or replace it at your expense.
- Don't expect other people to clean up after you; keep your work area neat and orderly so it doesn't become an eyesore for others.
- Don't display risqué calendars, posters, or other personal items that might offend someone else.
- Listen when other people are talking and don't interrupt them.
- When riding on an elevator with patients on carts or in wheelchairs, protect their privacy and don't stare at them.

PERSONAL ETIQUETTE

- RSVP to party invitations in plenty of time to let the host know if you'll be attending.
- Don't bring children or other guests with you to an event unless they've been invited.
- Acknowledge gifts by sending the giver a written thank-you note within 2 weeks.
- When seated for a meal, don't start eating your food until everyone at your table has been served; don't leave the table until everyone has finished eating.

- Refrain from texting and using cell phones during meals.
- When speaking on the phone, lower your voice to avoid annoying the people around you.
- When walking down the street or up or down the stairs, stay to the right.

PROFESSIONAL AND BUSINESS ETIQUETTE

- Shake hands with a firm grip when you meet someone; be aware that some people will resist a handshake because of an injury or concern about spreading germs.
- Refer to an older person or a superior (such as your boss's boss) by his or her last name (Mr. Smith rather than Bill).
- Respect other people's time and don't make them wait on you.
- When you put people on hold on the telephone, check back every few minutes to let them know you haven't forgotten about them.
- When people arrive for a meeting, if possible, offer them a beverage.
- Don't text, check e-mail messages, or talk on your cell phone when you're in meetings or with people who expect to have a conversation with you.
- Maintain eye contact when speaking with people; when speaking to a group, make eye contact with everyone, not just one person.
- When invited as a guest to eat with your supervisor or a coworker, don't order expensive menu items.
- When going through a buffet line, leave enough food for those in line behind you.

MANNERS

- When you notice someone carrying a heavy or cumbersome package, offer to help.
- When in a crowded area, offer your seat to an elderly or handicapped person, a pregnant woman, or anyone else who needs the seat more than you do.
- Hold doors open for people who are entering or leaving the building right before or after you.
- If an elevator is crowded, step back and wait for the next one.
- When encountering a disfigured or handicapped person, don't stare or ignore the person; make eye contact and acknowledge their presence in a friendly manner.
- Always say "please" and "thank you" and acknowledge the kindness of other people.
- Cover your mouth and nose when you sneeze; wash you hands frequently during flu season to reduce the spread of germs.
- Acknowledge people when they walk into the room and make them feel welcome.

There are far too many examples of polite behavior to list them all here. If you feel you need to learn more about courtesy, etiquette, and manners there are many good books available on the subject.

Teams and Teamwork

Your relationships with coworkers become even more important when working on teams, and teamwork is "the name of the game" in health care. In fact, many health care providers now rely on "high performance work teams" to care for patients and complete other assignments. Depending on your profession and where you work, you'll probably participate on many teams during your career.

Types of Teams

There are at least six different kinds of teams in health care. Some are based on disciplines that relate to different kinds of occupations and workers, such as radiographers, medical technologists, or unit secretaries. Some teams are composed of people from within the same department (*intra* means *within*) while other teams are composed of people from different departments (*inter* means *across*).

INTRADISCIPLINARY TEAMS

- People from the same discipline (radiography, for example) with similar educational backgrounds, job duties, and scopes of practice who work in the same department or different departments (main radiology, emergency department, outpatient radiology, etc.)
- A team of radiographers who might work together to select some new diagnostic imaging equipment and prepare for installation and staff training

INTERDISCIPLINARY TEAMS

- People from different disciplines, with different educational backgrounds, job duties, and scopes of practice and who work in the same department or different departments
- A team of medical technologists, phlebotomists, and nurses who might work together to coordinate the collecting, labeling, and processing of patient blood samples

INTRADEPARTMENTAL TEAMS

- People from the same department or work unit but with different educational backgrounds, job duties, and scopes of practice
- Surgical nurses, surgical technologists, and instrument technicians who might form a team to improve instrument sterilization and packaging

INTERDEPARTMENTAL TEAMS

- People from different departments, with different educational backgrounds, job duties, and scopes of practice
- Representatives from the information technology, admitting, and patient registration departments who might meet to streamline patient registration processes

There are at least two other types of teams in health care.

WORK TEAMS

- Meet on an ongoing basis as part of their jobs; a group of paramedics who might meet weekly to monitor patient transport and quality outcome data

PROJECT TEAMS

- Meet for a specified period of time and disband when their project has been completed; some projects are short term (creating a new electronic form for patient billing) while others are more long term (creating a new computerized database to track patient discharges)

Labeling your team isn't necessary but it's important to participate as an effective team member. High-performance work teams often work independently with little direct supervision. Management creates the team, identifies the members, arranges meeting times, communicates expectations, and clarifies the team's assignment. Then the team takes over:

- Arranging their own work schedules and holiday coverage
- Selecting new equipment and medical supplies
- Monitoring and improving quality outcomes
- Resolving budgetary and staffing issues
- Interviewing and selecting new team members

Team members may evaluate the performance of their teammates using 360-degree feedback performance evaluations. With responsibilities such as these, you can see why effective communication skills are so important. Team members can also benefit from extra training in group dynamics, negotiation, delegation, resolving conflicts, and valuing **diversity** (differences, dissimilarities, variations).

Regardless of what types of teams you serve on, you will need to become skilled at leading and following. You'll probably find yourself in both roles from time to time, even within the same team. Shared leadership is becoming more common. Members rotate the leadership role over time or each team member takes the lead when the task to be completed falls within his or her area of expertise or interest.

Leading team members is not the same thing as supervising team members. In many situations team members are peers, so no one on the team reports to another person on the team. If one team member fails to complete his or her responsibilities, the whole team may suffer. In many health care settings, team performance is just as important (or more important) as individual performance. When the team performs well, each member is held in high regard. When the team fails, each member is held accountable.

Group Norms

It should be clear that when working on teams your success as an individual depends on the success of your team. Think about some of the teams you've participated on. Which teams worked well together and which ones didn't? Establishing **group norms** might help. Group norms are expectations or guidelines that team members agree to follow to help the team function smoothly over time. For example, team members may be expected to:

- Attend all meetings, arrive on time, and stay until the end
- Speak up, play an active role, and participate in decision making
- Respect the ideas and opinions of others
- Follow through on obligations and complete assignments on time
- Carry their share of the workload
- Share information openly
- Cooperate and provide assistance when asked
- Focus on solutions instead of problems
- Serve as leader and follower as needed

It's not unusual for employees who work in teams to crosstrain with one another. As multiskilled workers, these employees are capable of performing multiple functions, often in more than one discipline. For example:

- A housekeeper might be crosstrained to perform basic maintenance and repair duties.
- A nursing assistant might learn to draw blood and prepare specimens for laboratory analysis.
- A unit secretary might learn basic nursing assistant skills.
- A maintenance worker might acquire carpentry skills.

Multiskilled workers who participate on teams tend to be highly productive. They enhance convenience for patients and staff, add versatility and flexibility to the staffing plan, and save the company money in labor costs. Effective communication and team skills are vital when multiskilled workers interact with coworkers from different disciplines. Crosstraining has become routine among health care employers so it's likely you will encounter this concept at some point during your career.

Consensus

Regardless of the types of teams that you serve on, one of your biggest challenges will involve achieving **consensus** (decision that all members agree to support) when decisions need to be made. Consensus is more than just voting on different options and declaring "majority rules." With majority rules, there are winners and losers—the majority wins and the minority loses. The objective of consensus, however, is to arrive at a win-win solution in which no one feels like a loser. Through group discussion, team members try to find an option that everyone can support. As you might imagine, achieving consensus is much more difficult than just taking a vote. But operating by consensus to find win–win solutions is the foundation of good teamwork.

Developing effective team skills takes time, especially when you're working with diverse groups of people with different personalities, values, and communication styles. However, serving on a smooth-running, high-performing work team can be one of the most satisfying experiences you'll have as a health care professional. Let's examine how honing your communication skills can help.

Communication Skills

Unfortunately, treating your coworkers as customers and applying good etiquette and manners at work won't guarantee that you'll get along with everyone. In fact, you can pretty much count on some interpersonal conflict with the people you work with. Everyone is working in a stressful environment. When you're under pressure or feeling rushed, you don't always practice your best communication skills. Because of the diverse array of people you encounter, you can't help but experience some difficulty getting along with everyone. As mentioned previously, you don't have to be friends with your coworkers, and it is okay if you don't like everyone you work with. But you can't choose your coworkers and you can't change them either, so you have to find ways to get along with everyone. Good communication skills can be a big help.

Communication is a two-way process—messages are sent and received. Both sides of the process must work well to support good communication. Unfortunately, messages are frequently misunderstood. Communication breakdowns often occur because the person receiving the message isn't listening to the person sending the message. Good listening skills are vital. It's important to not only *listen* to someone but to also actually *hear* what the person has to say. Most of us need to improve our listening skills. Here are some ways to do so:

- Learn to listen carefully and concentrate on the message so that you fully understand the other person's point of view.
- Repeat what the person has said in your own words to make sure you received the message accurately.
- Don't "half-listen" to other person while you're thinking about how to respond; you may miss part of the message.
- Ask the other person for clarification when you don't fully understand what he or she is saying. Or ask the person to state the message again using different words.
- Observe the person's **body language** (nonverbal messages communicated by posture, hand gestures, facial expressions, and so on) to gather more information.

Body Language

Most of the messages that people send out are communicated nonverbally through body language. This includes facial expressions, gestures, eye contact, "rolling" of the eyes, posture, body movements, tone and loudness of the voice, and so forth. Body language often communicates more information and a greater accuracy of information than the actual words people use. You can convey your anger, disappointment, or frustration with someone without even saying a word. Slumping in your chair, cowering in the corner, or avoiding eye contact with the person with whom you are communicating are all behaviors that send out messages nonverbally.

When communicating verbally, here are some things to think about:

- Be clear and concise so that your listener can easily understand.
- Use words and terms that your listener is familiar with.
- Give examples as further explanation.
- Avoid frustration when the other person just doesn't seem to "get it." Restate your message using different words.
- If the conversation seems to be going nowhere, ask a third person for help.

Communication Styles and Conflict Resolution

You've no doubt heard the phrase "dealing with difficult people." Responding to **confrontation** (to face boldly, defiantly, or antagonistically), confronting

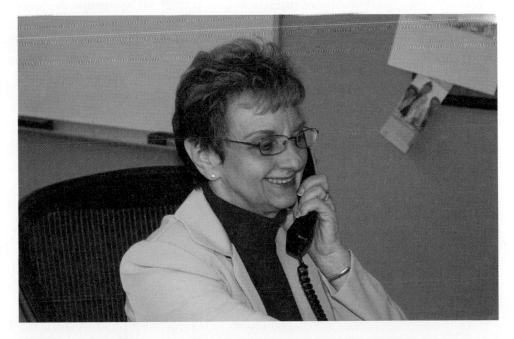

Figure 4-3 ■ **Facial expression conveys positive body language**

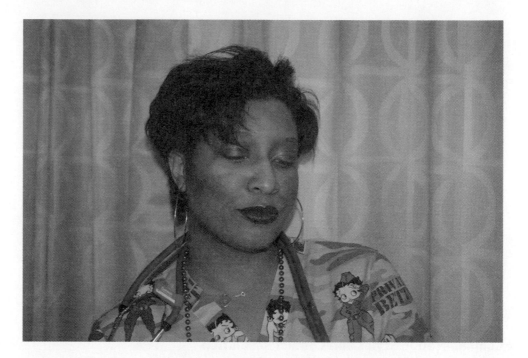

Figure 4-4 ■ Facial expression conveys negative body language

people yourself, and resolving interpersonal conflict all require some special communication skills in **conflict resolution** (overcoming disagreements between two or more people).

When you confront someone or respond to someone who has confronted you, the goal is to communicate your point of view in an open, honest, and direct manner. This means you are *open* to sharing your opinion, you are *honest* in stating your opinion, and you state your opinion in a *direct* manner to make sure the other person gets your point. Let's see how well these goals are met when using each of the four different styles of communication: aggressive, passive, passive-aggressive, and assertive.

Here's the scenario. You and a coworker both want Christmas off. Both of you have relatives arriving in town and wish to spend time with them. After discussing the holiday schedule, it becomes obvious that one of you must work, so you start the conversation.

AGGRESSIVE STYLE

In a loud, angry tone of voice you say, "I've worked here longer than you, so I get the day off! Besides, my kids are coming and they live farther away than your kids!"

Your coworker replies, "You got Thanksgiving off and I had to work! So I deserve Christmas off more than you! And besides, you don't have grandchildren and I do!"

You reply, "Why do you always have to insist on getting your own way? Every time we do the schedule, you complain!"

"I complain?" your coworker responds. "You're the one who always refuses to work overtime!"

You can imagine where the "conversation" goes from here. With aggressive communication, the conflict usually gets worse. You've expressed your opinion in an open, honest, direct manner. So why didn't the aggressive style of communication work? You failed to show respect or consideration for your coworker so he became defensive and fought back. Before long, anger took over, other issues entered the conversation, and the conflict escalated into an argument. Situations involving aggressive communication can turn violent, which might result in shouting or fistfights. The conversation might be overheard by other people including supervisors and patients. Did anyone "win" in this situation? Was the conflict resolved? It's clear the answer is "no." Let's try a different approach.

PASSIVE STYLE

In a meek, quiet tone of voice you say, "Well, I guess if you want Christmas off, I'll have to work. Maybe my kids can come back for Easter."

That was a pretty short conversation. Using passive communication, you failed to express your opinion in an open, honest, direct manner. You turned into a floor mat to be walked on. Your coworker won, he got his needs met, but you lost and came off looking (and feeling) weak and pitiful. Was the conflict resolved? Yes. But in the long run you'll resent your coworker and feel disappointed in yourself for not standing up for something that was important to you. Let's try again.

PASSIVE-AGGRESSIVE STYLE

You say, "Well, I guess if you want Christmas off, I'll just go ahead and work. Maybe my kids can come back for Easter." And then, as soon as you get the chance, you do something sneaky to "get even" with him. You send your supervisor an anonymous note saying your coworker takes longer breaks than he's supposed to. You spread malicious gossip about him behind his back. Or you call in sick on a busy day when the two of you are assigned to work together. After all, there are lots of ways to get even. Maybe getting even will make you feel better or maybe not. Using passive-aggressive communication, you still failed to express your opinion in an open, honest, direct manner. And to make matters worse, you did something sneaky and dishonest. Was the conflict resolved? No. Let's try one more time.

ASSERTIVE STYLE

In a normal tone of voice you say, "Well, we both want Christmas off. I'm sure you'd like to spend Christmas with your grandchildren. After all, you had to work Thanksgiving, didn't you? However, I've worked here twice as long as you so I have seniority. And my children are really looking forward to spending the day together as a family. So let's figure out a way to work this out so we can both get our needs met."

Maybe you could split the holiday shift. Maybe you could arrange a long weekend off to make up for one of you having to work the holiday itself. Maybe you could work together to find a third person who's willing to cover the holiday in exchange for a different day off. There is usually a workable solution to any problem but if you're arguing with the other person, your energy is spent on the conflict, not the solution. Using assertive communication, you stated your opinion in an open, honest, and direct manner and you did so in a way that showed respect and consideration for your coworker. Did it solve the problem? Maybe, maybe not. But assertive communication presents the best opportunity for you to work together, compromise, and come up with a solution that's acceptable to both of you. It's a win-win solution, which is the goal of conflict resolution.

It should be obvious that assertive communication is the only acceptable communication style at work. You must have enough self-respect to state your needs openly and honestly. You must not allow yourself to be "walked on," pitied, or tempted to do something underhanded and sneaky to get even. Professionals look out for themselves but do it in a way that shows respect for the needs and desires of their coworkers.

Assertive communication doesn't come easy—it takes practice. Maybe you're not used to standing up for yourself when someone confronts you or disagrees with you. Maybe aggressive or passive-aggressive communication has been your style up until now. If so, it's time to start working on a different approach that's more appropriate in the workplace. Put some effort into developing your assertive communication skills. Observe how other people deal with conflicts and the results they get. Then keep practicing your own skills. The more you practice, the easier it will become.

Learn to "choose your battles wisely." Decide which conflicts are really worth tackling and which you ones you should just "let go." Some battles aren't worth the effort. And be careful! Just because you're taking an assertive approach doesn't guarantee the other person will as well. Someone could turn aggressive on you. When communicating with a "difficult" person, make sure you can get out of the room quickly if you need to. If you have any concern about your physical safety, make sure there's someone else nearby who can come to your aid if necessary. Remember it can be a crazy world out there. You never know when someone might be carrying a weapon or behaving in an aggressive or passive-aggressive manner. Here are some things to think about when confronting someone:

- Treat the other person with respect. Give him or her the benefit of the doubt until you've fully investigated the matter.
- Make sure you have complete, accurate information before confronting someone. Don't proceed on assumptions or unverified, third-hand information that might not be true.

- Stay calm and keep your anger and tone of voice in check.
- Arrange a suitable time and place to discuss differences. Never conduct this type of conversation in a public area.
- Don't go off "half-cocked" only to later regret something you've said or done.
- Listen carefully and make sure you understand the other person's point of view.
- Aim for a win-win solution.
- Take safety precautions. You may be able to control your own behavior but you cannot control the behavior of the other person.

Once you fully understand the other person's point of view and he or she understands yours, there should be a middle ground where both of you can compromise and feel like your needs have been met.

When you have a conflict with a coworker, resolve it quickly. Procrastination only makes things worse. But calm down first and make some rational decisions about how to handle the matter. Attack the issue, not the person. Remember that you cannot change other people; only they can change themselves. All you can do is make your best effort at communicating appropriately. If necessary, ask another person with good conflict resolution skills to serve as an intermediary.

If one of your superiors is the "difficult person," proceed cautiously! Remember to respect his or her position of authority. Weigh the pros and cons of addressing the situation head-on or just learning to live with it. If you decide to discuss the matter with your superior, follow these steps:

- Plan in advance what you're going to say, how you're going to say it, and what response you'll give to how he or she might react.
- Practice delivering the message in advance and consider role-playing the situation first with someone you trust.
- Listen carefully, watch for a win-win resolution, and be open to receiving some constructive feedback that might help you form a more positive relationship with your supervisor in the future.
- If the matter is still unresolved and you cannot move forward, speak with a human resources representative or another person in authority in your department.
- If the situation is serious and cannot be resolved, you may need to transfer into another position.

Effective communication and conflict resolution skills will serve you well in all aspects of your life. Avoid letting other people "press your buttons." When you hear yourself saying, "She makes me so angry!" stop and think about that statement. You have a choice as to whether to be angry or not. Allowing other people to "make you" angry means you are handing over control of your behavior to someone else. Is that really what you want to do? Find ways to maintain control of your own behavior and don't allow other

CASE STUDY

It's been 6 weeks since Carla decided to report what she believed to be a conflict of interest on the part of the network's purchasing agent. And she's glad she did. An investigation uncovered several instances of dishonest behavior and the purchasing agent was fired. The network's director and Carla's practice manager thanked her for being attentive and willing to step up and report the wrongdoing of another employee. They told Carla they really appreciated what she had done to protect the reputation of the company and they said they wished other employees had a similar sense of loyalty and commitment.

Carla isn't sure if there's a connection to this whistle-blowing incident or not but she's just received a special assignment and a pay raise to go with it. She's now assigned to a brand new interdisciplinary team that's been formed to design and open a new clinic across town. Several coworkers have congratulated her and she suspects they're surprised that a relatively new MA could earn such an impressive assignment so quickly. But everyone seems to like Carla and she's been told she has great people skills, so she's happy about the change and looking forward to her new role.

But Carla's enthusiasm took a nosedive at the first team meeting. People were pulled from several different practices in the network to create the new team, so members were meeting each other for the first time. It became clear quickly that people had a lot of different opinions to share, which didn't surprise Carla. She had worked in health care long enough to know that nurses, medical assistants, physician assistants, office personnel, and doctors would have different perspectives and couldn't be expected to agree on everything, but the first meeting was chaotic. Several people tried to talk at the same time while others remained silent. No one was put in charge, so when three people tried to take the lead, conflict broke out. Some of the team members weren't very polite. They laughed at people's ideas and interrupted when others were trying to speak. One man became aggressive and left the meeting early.

Now Carla is worried. Her job depends on the team's success but some of the members don't seem up to the challenge. What should Carla do? Should she ask to be removed from the team, go back to her old job, and give up her raise? Should she take over leadership of the team and tell people to shape up? Is there something Carla could do to help the team function more effectively? What would you do if you were in Carla's place?

people to push you into doing things or saying things that you would rather not do or say.

There's obviously a lot to think about when communicating with people in person. Let's examine the many pitfalls of communicating with people electronically.

Electronic Communication

In today's highly technologic world, communicating electronically by e-mail, voicemail, texting, cell phone, Internet, telephone, and fax offers several efficiencies and convenience. However, electronic communication also creates the need for caution, especially when using e-mail, voicemail, and texting.

With e-mail and texting, the receiver sees only the words that you have conveyed. Without actually hearing you or seeing you, the message can become somewhat impersonal. The tone of your message (serious, humorous, etc.) could easily be misunderstood or misinterpreted by the receiver. You may have sent a humorous message but the receiver might think you were serious or vice versa. As mentioned previously, body language often conveys more information than the words used. Had you delivered your message in person, your body language would have communicated "humor," not "serious."

When delivering messages by voicemail, the receiver hears your words and your tone of voice but your body language is still invisible. When you need to be absolutely certain that your message has been conveyed and received accurately, it's best to speak with the person in person. The second best option is a live telephone conversation.

Another disadvantage of communicating by e-mail is accidentally sending a message to the wrong person or people. If you are a frequent user of e-mail, you've probably already made this mistake and hopefully learned a lesson. Either you mistakenly clicked on the wrong address, sent the wrong message to the wrong person, or forwarded a previous message to another person without realizing what you were doing. Similar problems may occur with voicemail messages. Anyone who receives an e-mail or voicemail message from you can forward that message to someone else without your knowledge or permission. These types of situations can be highly embarrassing and may accidentally reveal sensitive, confidential information to people who should not have access to it.

When communicating electronically:

- Slow down and think about what you are doing.
- Keep your messages short and to the point.
- Omit information that could become problematic if it falls into the wrong hands.
- Exercise care when forwarding previous messages. Before you click on send, double-check the content of the entire message and confirm to whom it is being sent.

With e-mail messages:

- Avoid using caps (using caps conveys yelling).
- Think how the recipient might react to the font and use of bold and color.
- Don't use attachments with little dancing figures or pictures.
- Be sure to include a subject line, greeting, and closing.
- Avoid text message abbreviations and use spelling and grammar check before sending the message.
- Before sending a message, be careful with reply and reply all. Don't select reply all unless it's really necessary for everyone to receive your reply.

Electronic communication isn't foolproof. You can't always be certain the message was received and read. People receive scores of e-mail messages at work every day. Sometimes messages are deleted accidentally before being read. People may become overwhelmed and never open all of their messages. And some people who have e-mail accounts at work never use them.

Keep in mind that electronic communication leaves a documented trail of messages. If you're angry with someone and send an emotionally charged message by e-mail, text, or voicemail, the receiver has documented evidence of your communication and could use it against you. If you had had a live telephone conversation with the person or met with him or her in person, there would be no documentation unless someone recorded the conversation.

With both e-mail and voicemail, even if you have deleted a message, it's still retrievable electronically. Deleting electronic messages does not mean they are gone forever. Always stop and think before you send any electronic message. Do you really want to send a message when you are angry or emotionally upset? How would feel if your message ended up in the wrong hands?

Be especially careful about posting personal information on social networking sites such as Facebook, Twitter, blogs, or other places on the Internet. Once personal information or photos of you are out on the Internet, they can't be retrieved. Anyone who has access to your online information can manipulate the content and share your information with anyone they care to. So-called privacy settings aren't necessarily effective and way too many people are learning this lesson the hard way. Health care companies are instituting Internet social networking policies to govern their employees' use of these sites. Computer security is major issue in today's world. Protect the security of your passwords, don't share passwords with anyone, and avoid using the same passwords at work that you use at home. Many companies require employees to change their passwords on a regular basis. Security can be compromised so the potential exists that non-authorized people could gain access to your e-mail correspondence and your company's private and

Recent Developments

THE RAPID GROWTH OF SOCIAL MEDIA

Communicating via social media is growing rapidly and becoming an integral part of people's lives around the world. Social media is the number one activity on the web. Half of the world's population is under 30 years of age and 96% of them use social media. About half of all baby boomers belong to at least one social media network. Recently, Facebook added two million users in less than 1 year. If Facebook were a country, it would be the third largest in the world. More than 1.5 million pieces of content are shared and 60 million status updates occur on Facebook each day. The fastest-growing segment of Facebook users is 55- to 65-year-old women. YouTube is the second largest search engine in the world with more than 100 million videos.

confidential information. Be sure to follow company policies that protect the security of computer systems and confidential information. Failure to do so could result in a breach of confidentiality, a violation of HIPAA and the HITECH Act laws, and embarrassment for you and your employer.

Written Communication and Presentation Skills

So far, we've focused on verbal, nonverbal, and electronic communication. Let's finish this discussion with a brief look at written communication and presentation skills.

Some jobs rely on written communication skills more than others but most everyone can benefit from sharpening their writing skills. Even if your job doesn't involve extensive writing, how you express yourself through written communication still has an effect on your work and your reputation. Poor written communication skills can impede advancement in your career. Here are some things to consider:

- If you struggle with writing, spelling, or punctuation, get some help. Take a course, do some self-study, or work one-on-one with a basic skills instructor.
- Make sure you can record accurate telephone messages, write notes to coworkers and your supervisor, and construct basic memos and letters should the need arise.
- If your job involves recording data on charts or other forms, make sure your writing is legible and your entries are accurate.
- If writing reports or preparing handouts for meetings is part of your responsibility, you'll need some higher-level writing skills to help you organize information and present it in an appropriate format. Make sure your computer skills include word processing.
- Don't use text messaging abbreviations in your written communication at work.

Spelling is important, especially in health care. With medical terms, changing just one letter in a word can change the entire meaning. If you fill out forms to order tests or treatments for patients, order patient supplies, or process bills or other kinds of paperwork, make sure you can spell terms correctly.

Few challenges in life are more anxiety producing than having to get up in front of a group of people and make a presentation. But public speaking skills are important, especially if your job requires you to give updates at meetings, make announcements to the rest of the staff, or teach coworkers something new. Becoming comfortable with public speaking is like facing any other fear—the more you do it, the better you'll get, and the more comfortable it will become. Start out small, with a group of supportive people, and build from there. Make sure you're well prepared, organized, and familiar with subject matter. Learn as much about your audience in advance as you can and tailor your presentation to meet their needs. Expect questions and comments; have your responses in mind. It's okay to admit that you're nervous. Most of the people in the audience will be glad it's you in front of the group instead of them.

For More Information

Etiquette and Manners
Emily Post
www.emilypost.com
802-860-1814

Public Speaking Skills
Toastmasters International
www.toastmasters.org
949-858-8255

Conflict Resolution
Association for Conflict Resolution
www.acrnet.org
703-234-4141

REALITY CHECK

How well you interact with other people is where "the rubber meets the road" in health care. From the first day you walk in the door to begin your new job, your people skills will be front and center. You might be the highest-skilled person in your entire company when it comes to the hands-on, technical skills of your job, but if you fail to form and maintain effective working relationships with your coworkers, your high degree of competence will soon be overshadowed by your lack of interpersonal skills. If you get labeled as a loner, troublemaker, or complainer, other people won't want to work with you and your supervisor will regret hiring you. Once this happens, you'll need to either change your ways or change your job and start over again.

Complying with etiquette standards and using good manners isn't difficult. In fact, treating other people in a polite, considerate manner should just be common sense. The problem is common sense isn't common anymore. Too many people have forgotten the lessons they learned as children and became adults who are totally focused on themselves. If you want to succeed in health care, you have to put the needs of other people ahead of your own. It's not about you. It's always about the patient—no matter what your job involves.

Key Points

- Work hard to develop and maintain positive relationships with other people.
- Consider coworkers your internal customers and treat them with kindness and respect.
- Display a friendly attitude, cooperate with people, and create a positive work environment.
- Be inclusive and welcome people into your group.
- Treat others as you want to be treated yourself, or better yet treat people the way *they* want to be treated.
- Show loyalty to your coworkers and your employer.
- Practice good etiquette and manners and treat everyone with courtesy.
- Develop effective team skills and use group norms when necessary.
- Strive to achieve consensus when making group decisions.
- Be aware of body language and the nonverbal messages you send.
- Listen carefully to make sure you hear and understand what's being said.
- Hone your assertive communication skills and use them to resolve conflicts.
- Use caution when communicating electronically
- Sharpen your written communication and presentation skills.

Learning Activities

Using information from Chapter Four:
- Answer the Chapter Review Questions.
- Respond to the What If? Scenarios.
- Complete Chapter Four activities on the website.

Chapter Review Questions

Using information presented in Chapter Four, answer each of the following questions:
1. Discuss the concept of interdependence and list three ways to strengthen relationships at work.

2. List two ways to demonstrate loyalty to your coworkers and two ways to demonstrate loyalty to your employer.

3. Identify two types of workplace teams and give an example of each.

4. Define the term *inclusive* and give two examples.

5. Explain the role of courtesy, etiquette, and manners in the workplace.

6. Define *consensus* and explain why it's important, but difficult, to achieve.

7. List three problems that may occur when communicating electronically and describe three ways to prevent them from happening.

8. Define *conflict resolution* and explain its importance.

9. Name the four styles of communication and describe the potential impact of each style.

10. Identify which communication style is most effective in conflict resolution and explain why.

What If? Scenarios

Think about what you would do in the following situations and record your answers.

1. Your supervisor has given you a project to complete. There's no way you can possibly get it done by yourself in time to meet the deadline. Your coworkers have expressed willingness to help, but you're used to working alone.

2. Three coworkers approach you, angry about a new policy. They're rounding up support to complain to management and want you to get involved.

3. A new person joins your work group. She's much older than everyone else and no one seems to like her. It's time to go to lunch and your coworkers leave her behind.

4. At an employee recognition dinner, the head of your company calls you to the stage to praise you for creating a new inventory tracking system. Although three of your coworkers helped you a lot, their names aren't mentioned.

5. Your company offers a six-month, part-time equipment repair course free of charge to employees. Those who enroll get to attend the classes on paid time. The company also pays the fee for course graduates to become certified as equipment repair technicians. After completing the course and becoming certified, you spot a newspaper advertisement recruiting certified equipment repair technicians for a company that competes with your employer and pays more.

6. You've been on call the last two weekends and it's your turn to be off. At the last minute, a coworker asks if there's any way you could take call for her this weekend. Her brother was seriously injured in a car accident and needs her help taking care of his children for a couple of days. You don't have any plans yourself, but you've already taken call two weekends in a row.

7. One of your coworkers is really beginning to annoy you. He takes longer breaks than he's supposed to and seems to disappear when there's work to be done. This morning, he kept a patient waiting for 20 minutes while he made several personal phone calls. When you remind him he has a patient waiting, he says, "Mind your own business! I'll get to him when I'm ready!"

8. You hear through the grapevine that a coworker has been spreading gossip about you. You're so angry that, as soon as she walks in the room, you're anxious to tell her just what you think of her behavior.

9. One of your coworkers is on corrective action for misspelling several medical terms on patient records. Unless she passes a medical terminology test by the end of the month, her job could be in jeopardy. She's lost her confidence and isn't sure if she can do it.

10. Your teammate finds out that you expressed doubts about his competence on a recent 360-degree performance evaluation initiated by his supervisor and now he wants to speak with you. You value your relationship with him but you're leaving on vacation early tomorrow morning and you're in a hurry to get home. Your teammate has already left work for the day. Sending him an e-mail message from home tonight would be the quickest way to explain your input on his performance evaluation.

PEARSON
myhealthprofessionskit™

Go to www.myhealthprofessionskit.com to access the Companion Website created for this textbook. Simply select "Basic Health Science" from the choice of disciplines. Find this book and log in using your username and password to access video scenarios, self-assessment quizzes, and more.

Cultural Competence and Patient Care

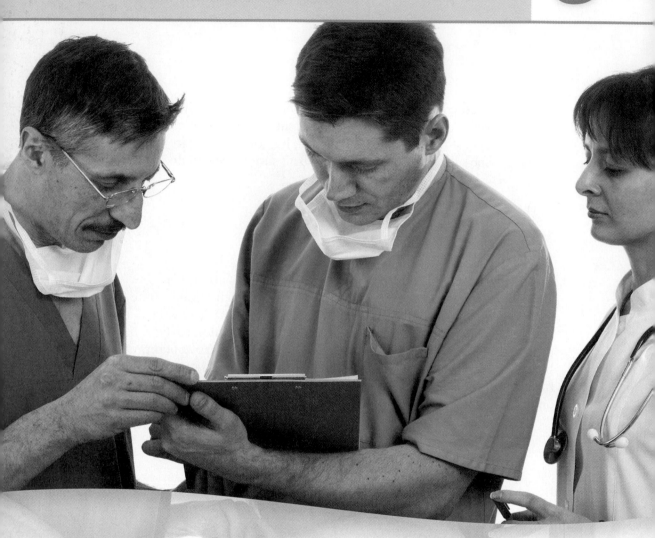

"How far you go in life depends on your being tender with the young, compassionate with the aged, sympathetic with the striving and tolerant of the weak and strong. Because someday in life you will have been all of these."

George Washington Carver,
Agricultural chemist, 1861–1943

CHAPTER OBJECTIVES

Having completed this chapter, you will be able to:

- Give three examples of diversity in addition to age and gender.
- Define the term *culture* and give three examples.
- Define the terms *bias* and *disparities* and explain how bias can result in health care disparities for members of minority cultural groups.

- Explain why health care workers need to be culturally competent.
- Give two examples of generational differences and describe how they might affect someone's work.
- List four types of health care customers.
- Describe how hospitals are measuring and reporting patient satisfaction.
- Describe five ways to provide good customer service for hospitalized patients and their visitors.

KEY TERMS

apps
biased
comparative data
cultural
    competence
culture
data mining

discrimination
disparities
empathetic
extenders
extroverts
first responders
generalizations

H-CAPS/HCAHPS
healing
    environment
introverts
invasive
mortality rate
non-compliant

norms
political correctness
prejudice
smartphone
stereotypes
telerobotics
transparency

Diversity and Culture

One of the challenges in forming effective working relationships is getting along with people whom you might see as different from you. You're probably familiar with the term *diversity* as it relates to racial differences (Caucasian, Black, Asian, etc.). Diversity also includes other kinds of differences based on cultural influences such as gender, age or the era in which you grew up, ethnic background, sexual orientation, religious beliefs, socioeconomic status, physical or mental conditions, occupation, neighborhood, family size, language, and more.

Culture is formed when groups of people share the same values and **norms** (expectations or guidelines for behavior). We all belong to multiple cultural groups at the same time. Depending on the situation, different cultures may take priority. For example, while you may belong to a large, rural, religiously focused family who holds well-established values about education and professionalism, your generational cultural norms might take priority over your religious culture when deciding how to dress appropriately for work.

Cultural groups share values and beliefs about what's most important to them. People in the nursing culture, for example, value disease prevention and keeping their patients safe. Cultural norms are the rules that members accept as normal: "the way we do things around here." These rules are learned (taught) and aren't usually written down but they're well understood by members of the cultural group. Members of each cultural group instill the norms about their values by way of customs, rituals, use of language, rewards and punishment, and modeling appropriate behaviors. Behaviors by individuals of the cultural group vary yet fall in line with the norms. (Indeed, there is more diversity within a cultural group than between cultures.)

How do values, norms, and behaviors influence a particular cultural group? Let's take a look at the value of "respecting your body and health." Some of the norms or rules that apply to "respecting your body and health" might include: focus on disease prevention, follow sound medical advice, eat nutritious food, exercise regularly, and avoid smoking. Although members of the cultural group share the same core value ("respecting your body and health") and understand the common norms, individuals will follow the norms with various behaviors. For example, using the *value* of respecting your body and the *norm* of eating nutritious food might mean *behaviors* of eating only organic for some, vegetarian for other individuals, or a mixture of lean protein and veggies with treats of high-fat, sugary desserts for others.

Why is it important to understand the difference among values, norms, and behaviors? Because it's easy to make judgments about other people based on their behaviors when you filter those behaviors through your own "cultural norms." You can't always identify other people's values or norms by their behaviors. This is where the cultural problem occurs. Once you start making judgments about other people, your decisions as well as your actions can become **biased** (favoring one way over another, based in having had some experience). Research shows that biased decision making by health care professionals can lead to **disparities** (lack of similarity or equality) in how members of minority cultural groups may receive health care services. When such disparities occur, patients may encounter unfair and misdiagnosed care and treatment.

Let's apply an example of how these concepts can play out at work. When you have a patient who doesn't take her prescription drugs as directed, you might label her as **non-compliant** (refusing or failing to follow instructions) and assume that she doesn't care about her body or her health or preventing disease. Perhaps you come from a medical culture in which taking a prescription drug is readily accepted and you would expect the patient's behavior to be in line with that (your) "norm." However, the patient who may not take the prescription drug as directed *does* value her body and her good health. She may have had a cultural upbringing with a norm of avoiding taking drugs of any kind. So when her behavior includes failing to take her prescription drugs as advised, her behavior is falling in line with her cultural norm, *but not yours*. You know that her condition would be greatly improved with the medication. Tension can creep into the interaction. You're working hard and have given her reliable advice and direction that really would help. From your point of view, she is resistant, noncompliant, and unreasonable in her rationale for not taking the drug. So in response you may have a tone of impatience, may disregard her preference for considering holistic solutions, may work with her a bit less, and may even blame her at some level for her condition. You may even disregard symptoms of something else because she has already demonstrated not complying with medical advice (even though the other symptoms may not need a prescription-related treatment). Actions are taken (or avoided) based on cultural differences and a disparity has occurred. Yet the patient shares the same value as you of caring about her health, demonstrating that behaviors are unreliable in assessing a person's values.

When cultural tension arises, it is usually because of different expectations around the cultural norms, not the values. When there is cultural tension, what can you do?

- Examine the assumptions about the behaviors relating to values; look to discover how the norms differ. Learn to accept different sets of cultural norms.
- Focus on discovering the core values you and the other person share. Finding the shared value can lead to a deeper understanding of the cultural dynamics and the resulting behaviors, and lead to different solutions.
- Mutually work toward behavioral change with more collaboration because the values have not been challenged.

Think about it. Would you want someone else trying to change your values? No, of course not. But if you realize that you both have similar values and you both might need to change your behaviors or expand your cultural norms to get a good result, it might be easier to find ways to work together

Cultural Competence

Cultural competence, the ability to interact effectively with people from different cultures, is crucial for health care workers. Cultural competence is a process of continual learning by being open to how their cultures influence people. Become confident in your ability to manage your responses to different cultures, including your own cultures. Cultural competence supports teamwork and helps ensure that decisions about patient care are made in an ethical and unbiased manner.

Cultural competence is not about **political correctness** (eliminating language or practices that could offend social sensibilities about cultural groups such as race and gender). When you encounter conflict that is caused by cultural differences in behaviors and norms, try to find the core value behind the norm. Once you've identified the core value that people share, focus on this common ground to help resolve the conflict. Here are some key strategies:

- Examine your own cultural norms first. Be aware that you experience other cultures through your own filters. Accept multiple approaches to "the way we do things around here."

- Be prepared to adjust your filters. If you don't understand another person's culture, ask him or her to share some information. Listen for understanding rather than defending "your" way.
- Your goal isn't to avoid judgment or **prejudice** (a judgment or opinion formed before the facts are known). Your goal is to acknowledge that judgment and prejudice exist and to learn to manage them. Remember that judgment and prejudice are thoughts that can be changed before taking action.
- Expose yourself to cultures that are different from yours. Stay, even if you feel uncomfortable. Discomfort is a sign that you're learning something.
- Learn to distinguish between **stereotypes** (beliefs that are mainly false about a group of people) and **generalizations** (facts, patterns, and trends about groups of people that are backed up by statistics and research findings).

Cultural competence occurs on a continuum:

- Unaware (truly unaware of a cultural situation)
- Denial ("Oh that doesn't really happen." Or, "What? I thought that ended years ago.")
- Defensiveness, defending one's own position as "the right one" ("Oh, yeah, well that's not as bad as what has happened to me or my people." "If your cultural group would work harder, you would be able to live like us.")
- Repulsion ("How could they live like that?" Or, "There's no way I could accept those people.")
- Pity ("If only they would … they could improve their lives." Or, "It's so sad those people live they way they do. It's too bad their lives aren't more like mine.")
- Minimization ("I don't care if someone is black or pink or green.") This minimizes the impact that color or some other characteristic may have had on a group of people because of the dominant social structure.
- Tolerance ("Do I have to put up with this person or group of people?")
- Admiration ("I admire people from. . . . cultural group. They've had to fight hard for justice.")
- Acceptance (Recognizing that diversity exists and appreciating the benefits that diversity brings)
- Inclusion and Integration (Recognizing the essential nature of diversity and actively seeking ways to include and integrate diversity; advocating for diversity)

Think about where your cultural competence lies on this continuum and adjust your filters and behaviors accordingly. Be aware that in every new situation, you may be in a different stage of competence. Listen to your own thoughts to get a sense of your attitude and cultural perspectives. When you feel like someone is being hypersensitive, research historical events that may have had a lasting impact on that person's cultural group.

Applying these concepts at work is really important because you need a variety of people with diverse perspectives to get the work done. If you're developing a new policy for your department, for example, you might look at the situation differently than a coworker who is much younger or older than yourself. A single woman might have a different perspective than a married man. Someone from a Mexican culture might place a greater value on a particular issue in the policy than someone from a Brazilian culture. An entry-level employee with life experience may offer different valuable insights than a seasoned, formally educated professional. All points of view must be taken into consideration to accommodate our diverse workforce. Let's start by examining differences in personality preferences.

Personality Types

Just as you are a unique person with your own personality and individual preferences, so are the other people with whom you come in contact. Personality types vary widely and they influence how people interact with one another and how they participate (or don't participate) in a group setting. Personality types also influence how people size up situations, make decisions, and approach their work.

Learn as much as you can about your own personality type and gain some insight into the personality types of the people with whom you work. There are many personality assessments available.

The Myers-Briggs Type Indicator (MBTI) is based on C. G. Jung's psychologic theories about how people differ in perception and judgment. Perception is how people become aware of things and take in new information. Judgment is how people arrive at conclusions based on what they have perceived. The MBTI focuses on eight sets of preferences and identifies 16 different personality types based on those preferences. For example, some people are **introverts** (people who focus on their inner world) while others are **extroverts** (people who focus on the outer world).

The Keirsey Temperament Sorter (KTS-II), based on Dr. David Keirsey's theory, describes behavior in one of four "temperament groups" with each group subdivided into four "character types." According to Dr. Keirsey, temperament is based on a combination of personality traits, behavioral patterns, values, and so on. Each temperament has its own characteristics. For example, some people talk about reality and everyday life—facts, figures, news, and so on. Other people talk about the abstract world of ideas, dreams, and beliefs. Some people behave in a practical manner that is focused on getting results. Other people behave in a cooperative manner that is focused on social interactions more than outcomes.

A third example is the Golden Personality Type Profiler, a workplace personality assessment that provides information to help explain why an individual behaves in a certain way in workplace situations. One of its five "global dimensions," tense versus calm, helps explain differences in how people respond to stress at work.

There is no right or wrong type on personality assessments—just different types. By becoming aware of your own personality type and the types of other people around you, you'll be in better position to understand differences and make the most of them.

Generational Differences

If you've had a job working with people from different age groups, you've probably already experienced some generational differences. Let's take a look at the characteristics of the four different generations found in today's workforce.

The Silent Generation (born between the 1920s and 1940s):

- Born during the Great Depression and World War II
- Believe in working hard, paying your dues, and clean living
- Value stability and security; resist borrowing and debt
- Don't like surprises; prefer clear lines of authority (reporting to one boss)

The Baby Boomers (born between the 1940s and 1960s):

- Largest generation on Earth; post–World War II baby boom
- Every life stage has been trend setting; their impact can't be ignored
- "If you have it, flaunt it" attitude
- Competitive, stylish, bossy, and curious
- Like shopping, leading, creating a vision; dislike paying debts and growing older
- Experienced a growing economy; plenty of job opportunities after college
- Staying in jobs and double Gen Xers in number so Gen Xers may have trouble "moving up the ladder"

Generation X (Gen Xers) (roughly born between the 1960s and 1980s):

- Unlike baby boomers, arrived almost unnoticed due to smaller numbers and less attention by the media
- Experienced a fading economic boom; saw their parents struggle with employment
- May have been "latch-key kids" who are independent, figure things out on their own
- Cynical generation; invented the term *whatever* . . .
- Come from broken homes and divorce common; may have been raised by two sets of parents
- Value friends, relationships, and loyalty
- Caught in the middle of economic change and companies in transition
- Naturally impatient; thrive on change
- Expect to be respected but it may take time before they develop respect for other people
- Like surprises, fun, and humor at work; dislike being micromanaged

Generation Y (born between the 1980s and 2000s):

- Arrived when society and the media were focused on babies and children

- Grew up with technology so it comes natural to them
- Want to get involved and make the world a better place
- Caring, honest, optimistic, clean-cut
- Like shopping, friends, family, the environment; dislike dishonesty and unbalanced lifestyles
- Respond to leaders who show integrity
- Like to be challenged, try new things, and learn in a hands-on manner
- Want to continually learn and expect the workplace to provide that opportunity
- Work isn't their life; they fit work into life and will leave an organization if work-life balance and growth aren't included

As you can tell by reading these descriptions, generational differences can have a big impact in the workplace. Think about the age groups of the people that you work with and how you can make the most of these generational characteristics. As you progress in your career and gain some leadership skills, familiarity with generational differences will become even more important as you figure out how to motivate, challenge, and reward each individual.

CONSIDER THIS

ONLINE RESOURCES AND SUPERCOMPUTERS

Patients are taking advantage of online resources to learn about medical conditions and compare prices and outcome statistics such as **mortality rate** (the ratio of deaths in an area to the population of that area, over a 1-year period) and readmission rates for local hospitals. This **comparative data** (information gathered from multiple sources that is analyzed to identify similarities and differences) allows patients and consumers to shop for health care services, providing more **transparency** (open, clear, and capable of being seen) among health care providers. As patients become more informed, they're playing a larger role in making decisions about their health care.

First responders (the first people to appear and take action in emergency situations) such as EMTs, paramedics, and flight doctors and nurses are using a **smartphone** (a mobile telephone that has advanced computing and connectivity features) with **apps** (software applications for smartphones and computerized hand-held devices) to access volumes of medical information on drugs, drug interactions, and treatment options whenever needed to speed up the care process before the patient arrives at the emergency department.

Researchers are using large computerized databases to store and analyze information on thousands of patients. Through **data mining** (sifting through large amounts of data to find significant information), they can follow patients before and after treatment to figure out which approaches work best. In the past, this type of research could take years but with today's supercomputers the analysis can be done in just minutes.

Occupational Cultures

In health care, another type of culture is the occupation in which you work. Registered nurses, for example, have a culture based on their educational background, where they work, what functions they perform, and the knowledge and abilities they possess. Physicians have a culture, too, as do medical technologists, maintenance workers, and so forth.

In health care organizations, there's a hierarchy based on these cultures and it sometimes causes problems. One example is **extenders** (people who assist other workers who are more highly educated and experienced). Patient care assistants, patient care technicians, and nursing assistants are examples of nurse extenders. Sometimes called *unlicensed assistive personnel*, these employees lack the training and credentials that RNs have but they work alongside RNs. Housekeepers and phlebotomists may also be assigned to work on patient care units. Sometimes extenders and other employees may have trouble fitting in and feeling like they're part of the team.

As mentioned previously, crosstraining has become common in health care. Since multiskilled workers are trained to function in more than one discipline, they often work in more than one area. They may encounter multiple cultures and might not feel totally accepted or comfortable in any one of them.

Health care teams are often composed of workers from different occupational cultures. Surgical teams, for example, include surgical technologists, surgical nurses, surgeons, and anesthesiologists. These teams are supported by schedulers, surgical attendants, instrument technicians, and others. Each type of worker has a different education level and scope of responsibility but all of them play important roles in the operating room.

Anytime someone "different" enters a group, he or she may experience difficulty fitting in and being accepted by others. This is a common problem when dealing with diversity. Do differences have to create difficult challenges? Is it really a problem if your coworkers are younger or older than you, of a different gender, or from a different race or ethnic group? Does it really matter if some have more education than you or less?

Everyone needs to work a little bit harder to get to know one another and figure out how to use differences to the group's advantage. The point is you're all there for the same purpose—to provide high-quality health care. Focusing on the mission of patient care gives diverse groups of workers some common ground to build on.

Diversity is an absolute necessity because the world would be a stagnant and boring place if everyone were alike. Health care professionals serve a diverse array of patients. Ideally, the health care workforce should be as diverse as the patient population so that workers can see things from the patient's point of view. This is why many health care companies try to recruit new employees who possess some of the same diverse characteristics as their patients.

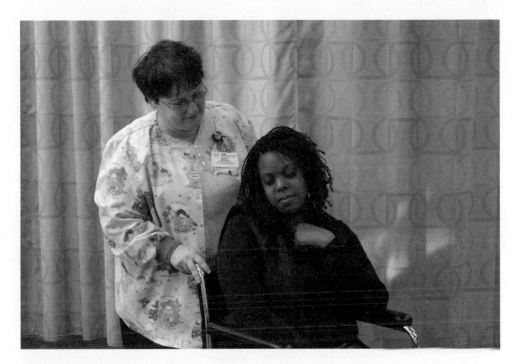

Figure 5-1 ■ **Worker escorting a wheelchair patient**

Respect

Diversity and respect go hand in hand. Regardless of whether you're working with people just like yourself or people who are different from you, respect is the basis for getting along well with everyone. Once you understand how people differ from one another and you realize there aren't "good people" or "bad people"—just "different people"—you can learn to respect everyone regardless of differences.

Much has already been said about the need to show respect for people but it's especially important to show your respect for employees who work in service and support roles such as housekeepers and food service workers. The health care culture places great value on its highly educated clinical care-givers such as registered nurses, doctors, and pharmacists, but lower-skilled workers often feel like they're at the bottom of the ladder, sometimes treated as if they're almost invisible. As a result, they may feel underappreciated and taken for granted. Take time to acknowledge their efforts and let them know that you value and respect the work they do.

The same is true for people above you on the occupational ladder. You may see highly educated people failing to give subordinates (including you) the credit they deserve. Try to give them the benefit of the doubt and don't take their lack of appreciation personally. When people function under stress, they don't always take time to thank other people for their efforts. Always respect authority. Even if you dislike your supervisor as a person, or you find fault with his or her job performance, it's still important to show respect for his or her experience and position within the organization.

Working with Patients

Most of what you need to know when working with patients will be covered in other classes that are directly related to your discipline and the types of patients with whom you will work. The remainder of this chapter will focus on patients as customers, exploring some of the factors involved in ensuring a high level of patient satisfaction. We'll also take a quick look at how to apply customer service standards when working with visitors, guests, vendors, and doctors—all of whom are considered customers of the health care industry. Depending on your job, you may deal with some or all of these different kinds of customers.

Before taking a closer look at customer service and the role it plays in patient care, let's examine patient rights and responsibilities.

Patient Rights and Responsibilities

Working with patients requires a partnership between the patient and his or her caregivers. Regardless of where patients go to receive health care services, they have certain rights that must be protected by health care personnel. For example, patients have the right to:

- Be treated with respect and without **discrimination** (unfair treatment of a person or group on the basis of prejudice), regardless of their medical condition, socioeconomic status, or other factors
- Privacy of their medical records
- Make a treatment choice (know their options and make the choice that's best for them)
- Informed consent (understanding the risks and benefits before agreeing to a test or treatment)
- Refuse treatment
- Make end-of-life decisions (use or nonuse of feeding tubes or ventilators to prolong life)

  Patients also have responsibilities. For example, patients should:

- Be honest with their health care providers (disclose information about their habits and their health)
- Comply with treatment plans (take medications as prescribed, for example)
- Show respect for their providers (keep appointments, show up on time, etc.)
- Fulfill financial obligations

RECENT DEVELOPMENTS

LESS-INVASIVE SURGERY

Surgery is becoming less **invasive** (an assault or attack) due to laser procedures and miniature cameras that allow surgeons to perform operations with very small incisions. Less invasive procedures are leading to less scarring, shorter recovery times, less hospitalization, and more patients eligible for the treatments. Surgical robots such as Da Vinci are becoming more routine.

Using **telerobotics** (robots controlled from a distance using wireless connections; used in conducting remote surgery), scientists are now developing tiny robots that can be inserted into the patient's mouth or nose to help perform surgical procedures without making an incision. Robots crawl and swim, taking pictures as they move around. With ARES (Assembling Reconfigurable Endoluminal Surgical System), after the patient swallows 15 separate parts, the robot self-assembles the parts inside the body to help surgeons complete the procedure. With SpineAssist, a tiny robotic fly controlled by a magnet outside the body travels through arteries and veins, detecting blockages and delivering drugs directly to tumors. More of these amazing new devices are on the way.

Customer Service

Some people cringe at the thought of referring to patients as *customers* but health care is a business and patients are the customers. It's important that health care customers are pleased and satisfied with the services they receive.

So much of what is being done to improve patient care relies on technology but it's important to remember that health care is a hands-on service industry where "high touch" is just as important as "high tech." Supercomputers and medical robots have their place but technology can never replace the human element when it comes to caring for patients.

Similar to your coworkers, your patients are a highly diverse group of people. They represent all personality types and a wide variety of differences. Some will be easy to get along with, others will be more difficult, and some will be downright nasty. Some patients will appreciate your efforts while others will not. But they all deserve to be treated with respect and good manners. Applying what you've learned so far in your interactions with patients is where "the rubber meets the road." Remember the difference between hard skills and soft skills? Everyone expects you to be competent (hard skills)—that's just a given. What will set you apart as a professional is how you behave (soft skills).

Working in direct patient care is a privilege. It's an honor to have other people entrust their health and safety to you. It's also an awesome responsibility. Today's patients have high expectations regarding how they will be treated by health care workers and they have choices as to where to obtain

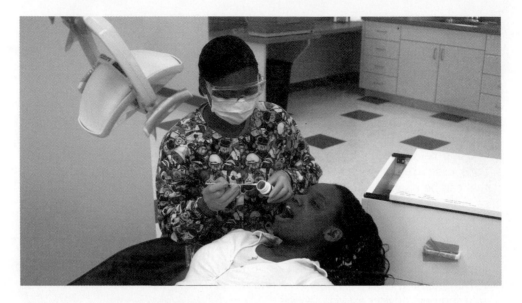

Figure 5-2 ■ Patient undergoing a dental procedure

health care services. Patients won't hesitate to go someplace else for their care if they believe they haven't been treated well. Dissatisfied patients will complain to their doctors and before long, the doctors will start referring their patients elsewhere.

When patients have a decision to make about where to go for their health care, they assume that most, if not all, of the hospitals and doctors in town provide quality care. What differentiates one health care provider from another often comes down to customer service—the patient's experience. As a result of this increasing focus on customer service, patient satisfaction has become a top priority. Patient satisfaction is now carefully measured and tracked over time. Many health care companies are providing customer service training for their employees and starting "service excellence" programs to raise their patient satisfaction scores.

Patient Satisfaction

Many hospitals have been collecting patient satisfaction data for their own internal use but until the **H-CAPS** survey was recently introduced, there was no standard approach for all hospitals to use in collecting this data and sharing it with the public. Also known as **HCAHPS** (Hospital Consumer Assessment of Healthcare Providers and Systems), the survey asks 27 questions to collect data about the patient's perception of the quality of his or her hospital experience. The survey is given to a random sampling of adult patients with a variety of medical conditions between 2 days and 6 weeks after they've been discharged from the hospital. The survey can be conducted by mail, telephone, or combination of the two. Questions solicit feedback regarding communication with the nurses and doctors, pain management, cleanliness, noise levels, details about medications, and so on. Patients are also asked to rate the hospital overall and whether or not they would recommend the hospital to other patients. Interestingly, patients who are admitted into the hospital via the emergency department (ED) tend to give lower scores on satisfaction surveys. Since the percentage of patient admissions via the ED is somewhat high in many hospitals, extra efforts should be taken to meet or exceed the expectations of these types of patients.

HCAHPS focuses on creating a culture of "always"—always delivering quality care to every patient during every encounter. Since data collection methods are standardized and hospitals post their results on a public website (www.hospitalcompare.hhs.gov), patients and other stakeholders have access to meaningful comparative data. Public reporting of survey results provides incentives for hospitals to improve the patient experience and become more transparent in sharing their outcomes. Patient satisfaction data is expected to play a major role in health care reform because hospitals that fail to receive high marks for patient satisfaction will receive less financial reimbursement for services provided to Medicare patients. The federal government is gearing up to implement pay for performance or value-based purchasing as a way to encourage more high-quality, patient-focused care.

THINK ABOUT IT

HEALING ENVIRONMENTS

Green initiatives, which focus on protecting the environment, are leading hospitals and other health care organizations to create a more **healing environment** (a physical space designed to reduce stress, ensure safety, and uplift the spirits of patients, visitors, and staff) to benefit both patients and workers. Research has shown that the quality of the environment can improve the healing of patients and the morale and efficiency of staff. Calming spaces designed with carefully chosen colors, lighting, and building materials can lift the spirits of seriously ill patients and reduce the stress of busy health care workers. Green initiatives, which help save energy and reduce waste, are well timed since many health care organizations are gearing up to build new hospitals, clinics, and nursing homes to replace outdated facilities and respond to the increasing demands of the baby boomer population.

Developers are designing energy-efficient utility plants, improving waste management and recycling efforts, and incorporating recycled materials, natural sources of light, and live plants and trees.

Being There for Patients

When you work in direct patient care, the patient should be the focus of everything you do. It's not about you, your department, or your schedule for the day. It's *always* about the patient. When you arrive for work, remember this. Today is just another typical day for you. But for your patients, it could be a day that they will never forget.

Patients will tell scores of people about their experience and how they were treated. Patients don't miss much—they hear and notice everything going on around them. If there's tension among the staff, they pick up on it. If a piece of equipment doesn't work, the restroom hasn't been cleaned, or the lettuce on the cafeteria salad bar is rotting, they notice. Patients spend a lot of time (too much time) waiting. It's amazing how much information a patient can acquire just sitting in a waiting room or lying on cart headed for surgery. If you think the patient can't overhear your phone conversation down the hall, think again.

When people become patients, they're vulnerable and at their worst. They're in pain and anxious, worried, confused, and overwhelmed with the medical experience. Many patients feel helpless, having to turn themselves over to strangers who will make decisions about their care. They're concerned about what might happen to them, how their lives will be affected, how their children and spouse will fare in their absence, and a whole host of other issues. Patients need reassurance and confidence that they're in good hands. As mentioned previously, how you look, communicate, and behave can have a tremendous impact on their feeling of security.

Everything you say and do makes an impact on patients. A small act of kindness on your part may be huge to your patient. Patients tend to pick their favorite caregivers. Upon returning, they may ask to have the same person take care of them again. Some caregivers "go the extra mile" and those are the people whom you want your patients to remember. Think back to the discussion about "being present in the moment." You must be able to filter out everything else going on around you and concentrate on "being there" at that precise moment for that patient. The connections that professionals make with their patients are not the result of just acting or performing a duty. The ability to connect with patients is a reflection of the caregiver's personal values and professional priorities—an indication that caring for others comes straight from the heart. Isn't this the kind of person whom you would want taking care of you and your loved ones?

Remember what you've learned about valuing differences and diversity. These concepts apply to patients and your other customers, too.

- It's not your place to be judgmental. It doesn't matter if your patient is wealthy, poor, homeless, elderly, a transvestite, a celebrity, or a criminal. Each patient should receive the same level of respect, quality of care, and customer service.
- Protect your patients' dignity, self-respect, and personal possessions.

- Refer to patients as *Mr.* or *Ms.* instead of *honey, sweetie,* or *dear.* You may think calling someone *honey* is a sign of caring but keep in mind that many patients (and other customers) object to these kinds of terms.
- Be compassionate and **empathetic** (relating to another person's emotions and situation).

Anticipate your patients' needs and be prepared to meet them. No request or concern is too trivial. But if a patient asks you for a drink, food, medication, or help walking to the restroom, don't fulfill the request unless your job includes these duties. Always refer any matter that is outside of your scope of practice to the patient's nurse or another caregiver on the unit and make sure the appropriate person follows through.

When communicating with patients, use terms they can understand. If they ask you a question you aren't capable of answering or aren't authorized to answer, refer the question to the appropriate person. Here are some things to keep in mind to protect confidentiality:

- Never read a patient's medical record unless it's part of your job.
- Never divulge information about a patient's medical status to the patient's family members, clergy, or other visitors without the patient's permission.
- Confine the exchange of confidential information to a need-to-know basis when discussing patients with other health care professionals.
- If you have patients who are celebrities, leaders in your organization, or coworkers, make sure you protect their privacy and give them every consideration that you would give other patients.
- Never ask questions or make comments in a public area that might embarrass a patient or violate privacy. For example, a medical assistant should never raise his or her voice to ask Mr. Jones, who is sitting in the public waiting area, whether he remembered to bring his stool sample!
- Avoid the temptation to give your own personal opinion when a patient asks, "Which doctor in this group is the best?" or "Which doctor would you take your child to?"
- Don't discuss your own medical history or the medical histories of your family members with patients.
- Always stop and think—if *you* were the patient, how would you want to be treated?

Patient Visitors

No discussion of customer service would be complete without mentioning patients' visitors—their family members and close friends. Patients' families are their lifeline to their normal life. When patients invite other people to be a part of their medical experience, these other people become part of the patients' team. Remember that *family* may mean something very different to patients than to you. Accept whom they identify as family and help them become a part of the patients' team.

CASE STUDY

Carla was disappointed in how poorly her new team functioned during its first meeting so she found some books and other reference material on group dynamics, meeting facilitation, negotiation, and conflict resolution. When the team met for the second time, she wasn't the only member who voiced concerns about the need to work together more effectively. Carla had read about the concept of group norms and thought it made sense. She suggested that her teammates develop some group norms to serve as guidelines as they moved forward. Other people liked the idea and after about 30 minutes of discussion their "rules" were posted on the conference room wall for everyone to see and follow.

Carla was pleased that people liked her suggestion and relieved that the group was moving along more smoothly now. Several sub-committees had been formed to coordinate a series of projects. Over time, it was becoming apparent that Carla was emerging as a leader of her team. She realized that,

with practice, she was getting pretty good at facilitating the meetings. She made sure that everyone's voice was heard and their opinions were respected. She worked hard to improve her communication skills and develop stronger organizational and time management skills.

Carla's supervisor was very pleased with her performance as were other leaders in the network. As a result, Carla was appointed team leader of the new Patient Experience sub-committee created to figure out what it would take to deliver first-class customer service in the new clinic still under construction. Carla was thrilled and nervous at the same time. In addition to her current job, she had only worked in one other place and that was the small practice where she did her practicum. With only limited patient care experience, she had no idea where to begin in coming up with a plan to provide the best patient care experience of any clinic in town.

What should Carla do? What would you do if you were in Carla's place?

Patients need families and friends to help them through difficult situations. Having clergy present may help. Sadly, not all patients have a support system. Some patients will complete their entire hospital stay with no family or visitors present. These patients need some special compassion and attention from their caregivers. Other patients have large families and lots of friends and sometimes this can cause problems. Policies regarding hospital visiting hours have always been controversial. Some hospitals strictly enforce limited visitation while others have abandoned visitation limitations altogether. The problem is that visitors don't always use common sense. If a person is sufficiently sick or injured to require hospitalization, then he or she needs rest and shouldn't be overtaxed with too many visitors. However, maintaining connections with family and friends is an important part of the healing process. Sometimes it's up to the caregiver to enforce limitations on visitors to carry out the wishes of the patient and what's best for his or her recovery.

Families of seriously ill patients may literally "camp out" at the hospital. They want to be as close to their loved one as possible and for as much time as possible. Spouses may spend the night in their loved one's room, even though it's very uncomfortable. Families bring things from home to comfort the patient, such as favorite foods, flowers, and personal items. They may bring clothes and toiletries because they are "living there" for the time being. The patient's room could become cluttered with people and things. Try to avoid viewing this as an inconvenience to you and remember—this is patient and his or her family's "home away from home" for the time being. Providing family support is an important part of customer service and patient care.

As mentioned previously, patients notice everything. When patients are hospitalized for several days, they and their family spend hours and hours and days and days waiting. Their lives are on hold until their medical situation is resolved and they can resume their normal routine. With so much time on their hands, they notice when the free coffee down the hall isn't strong enough, the upholstery on the chairs is threadbare, and the elevator doors close too quickly. When it's finally time to eat, there's never an extra wheelchair available to push grandma down to the cafeteria. The patient's room is too hot or too cold. The meal tray was supposed to be delivered 20 minutes ago and when it finally arrived, the milk was white instead of chocolate. The TV remote control doesn't work the way it's supposed to.

Patients and families may become irritated when they don't get medical information about the patient's condition and treatment plans quickly enough. Doctors make rounds on the patient care units when it's most convenient for them. Families may stay in the room all day and refuse to leave even for meals for fear of missing the doctor when he or she makes rounds. They may pressure you for information that you don't have and ask for answers that you cannot give.

Patients who receive health care in outpatient settings are also on a quest for information. After seeing their doctor in his or her office and undergoing diagnostic tests, patients want to hear the results of those tests as quickly as possible. They also have questions about the results and next steps. All too often, patients receive a postcard in the mail or a brief phone call from the doctor's nurse or medical assistant directing the patient to pick up a prescription at the pharmacy. Patients may not have the opportunity to get all of their questions answered until returning for a follow-up doctor's visit several weeks later. If part of your job is calling patients to inform them of test results, have sufficient information at hand to answer their questions. Today's health care consumers are often well informed. They don't just want to hear, "Your results were slightly elevated." They want details and actual numbers so they can go online and learn more about their conditions and potential treatment options. In situations when you can't provide all of the information requested, don't be surprised if the patient asks to speak with the doctor.

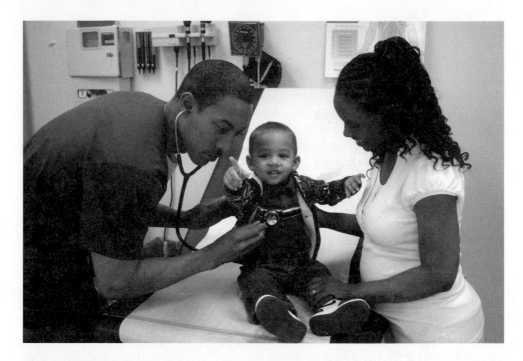

Figure 5-3 ■ Examining a pediatric patient

Some doctors willingly take phone calls while others may do so begrudgingly or not at all. Depending on your job, you may be in an assistant role to the physician, a liaison between the patient and his or her doctor. Do your best to meet the patients' needs while still working within your scope of practice.

Try to give your patients and their family members the benefit of the doubt and remember that their lives are in limbo. They're temporarily living in suspended animation, in some surreal world usually not by choice. They're uncertain about what's going to happen next and no one has all of the answers. Take a deep breath and remember why you went into health care. Give them some slack and rejoice that *you*, unlike your hospitalized patients, get to go home in a few hours.

Avoid the temptation to give personal advice or to express your own religious beliefs. When appropriate, generate some humor and laughter. Be positive whenever you can. Even tiny improvements in the patient's condition mean a great deal to the patient and his or her family members. Here's when your optimistic "the glass is half full" attitude can be helpful. Perhaps the patient's blood pressure and heart rate haven't settled down during the past hour but they haven't worsened either. Maybe the patient isn't well enough to be transported to radiology for a chest x-ray but he can sit up in bed and have a portable radiograph taken in his room. Maybe the patient's IV supply can't be completely disconnected but the dosage has been reduced. Look for things to be happy about and express them. Optimism and a positive outlook on the part of caregivers are important to patients. A positive frame of mind can lead to improvements in a patient's condition. When undergoing high-risk procedures, patients who are optimistic and more relaxed may have better outcomes. If a patient thinks his or her medical team has given up, he or she may give up, too, but don't give patients "false hope" or "get their hopes up" inappropriately. Some of your patients won't get better. Some won't leave the hospital alive.

Working in direct patient care is a privilege. You may be called upon to help prepare someone for death. The patient and his or her family will have difficult decisions to make. They will need privacy and time to talk, cry, and express their love and other emotions. They may have to "say goodbye" as the cart is wheeled out of the room on its way to surgery, facing the prospect of never seeing their loved one alive again. Those are the moments that your patients and family members will remember forever, and you are a part of it. Just as you may help usher in a new life you may also be present when someone passes. Both are humbling experiences that you cannot begin to imagine until you go through them yourself.

Working with Doctors, Guests, and Vendors

Doctors are customers, too. As with other customers, you will encounter doctors from various cultures, with different personality types and communication styles. You'll work with doctors whom you really like and respect and others whom you would avoid if you could. Some will take an interest in you, answer your questions, and explain procedures as they are performed. They'll "go the extra mile" for their patients and they'll express appreciation for their staff. Others may appear smug, dispassionate, indifferent, or downright rude. To save time, they may record information for the patient's medical record in front of the patient during an office visit rather than speak directly with the patient and then become irritated if the patient interrupts or asks a question. (Yes, unfortunately this really happens.) Some doctors may treat you as if you're invisible or unimportant. One day a doctor may be friendly and the next day he or she may be grumpy. A doctor may appear angry when speaking with you, yet his or her anger may actually have nothing to do with you at all.

Even though some doctors will be demanding and intimidating, try to keep in mind that doctors are just people, too. They have hopes and dreams, feelings and fears, frailties and flaws just like everyone else. Much of the time they're in a hurry and under a great deal of stress. Some of them literally hold life and death in their hands on a daily basis. Practicing medicine is an enormous responsibility and it takes its toll. Until you have walked in doctors' shoes, you have no idea what their jobs are like.

Occasionally a doctor may ask you to do something that's outside of your scope of practice. He or she may mistake you for a different type of worker or may not be familiar with your training and job duties. If this happens, speak up! Don't just go ahead and do something you aren't qualified to do because a doctor asked you or told you to. Say politely, "That's not within my scope of practice but I'll go get someone who can help you." If you are competent and apply your best communication and customer service skills, you'll likely get along just fine with the doctors.

Guests in your facility are also customers and they, too, are a diverse group of people. Some may be lost or stressed out, running late for an important meeting or a job interview. Others may be in the building to attend a conference or keep an appointment with someone in management. The most frequent request that you'll get from guests is help with directions. Here are some things to remember:

- If you work in a large building, make sure you know your way around so you can give good directions to other people.
- If you have the time or are headed in that direction anyway, offer to walk with people to make sure they get to their destination.
- If someone is waiting to see your supervisor or someone else in your area and you have access to coffee, water, or a soft drink, offer the person a beverage.
- If you know someone is going to have to wait for awhile, let the person know and explain why.

Do whatever you can to make guests comfortable. Your customers will appreciate even a small gesture of kindness.

The last group of customers is vendors, people who work for companies that your company does business with. Vendors might be salespeople from a patient supply company, insurance agents, drug company representatives, or people who work for advertising agencies or temporary services. Just like other customers, they too should be treated with respect, manners, and good customer service.

For More Information

Research on Cultural Competence in Health Care
Agency for Healthcare Research and Quality
U.S. Department of Health and Human Services
www.ahrq.gov (Type "cultural competence" in the search box)

MBTI Assessment
The Myers & Briggs Foundation
www.myersbriggs.org

Keirsey Temperament Sorter Assessment (KTS-II)
www.Keirsey.com
650-276-0770

Golden Personality Type Profiler
Personality Pathways
www.personalitypathways.com

Patient Satisfaction Scores (H-CAPS/HCAHPS)

Centers for Medicare and Medicaid Services (CMS)
www.cms.gov/HospitalQualityInits/30_HospitalHCAHPS.asp

Patient Satisfaction and HCAHPS Information

www.hcahpsonline.org

Hospital Compare Website

Provides public access to comparative data on patient perceptions of care and other quality metrics; helps consumers choose a hospital
www.hospitalcompare.hhs.gov

Patient Rights

The Patient Care Partnership: Understanding Expectations, Rights, and Responsibilities
American Hospital Association
www.aha.org/aha/issues/Communicating-With-Patients/pt-care-partnership.html
800-242-2626

REALITY CHECK

This chapter includes several terms and concepts that may be somewhat confusing—cultural competence, values, norms, behaviors, culture, discrimination, prejudice, disparities, political correctness, and so forth. Here's the bottom line. Learning to work with diverse groups of people will probably require a significant amount of time and experience before you begin to feel confident and competent. This is especially true if you've lived in a sheltered environment most of your life without experiencing people from many different cultures. If you expect to excel in your role as a health care professional, you must learn to not only get along with people who are different from you, but you must also learn to embrace differences and make them work to everyone's advantage.

Each time you encounter someone who is different from you, stop and think before you act. Are you judging this person based on your own cultural values and norms? If so, you're normal. It is human nature for people to judge other people based on their own values and prejudices, but don't allow these judgments to guide your behavior because the assumptions you've made about this other person might not be accurate. Remain open-minded and try to see things from the other person's point of view. If you find that difficult, ask the person for help. Most people enjoy talking about their background and the cultures in which they grew up and live. Don't hesitate to help other people learn more about you. Everyone has insights to share. You might be surprised what you'll learn.

Key Points

- Develop an appreciation for diversity and differences among people.
- Examine your own cultural norms and avoid letting bias and prejudice govern your behavior.
- Expose yourself to cultures that are different from yours and share information about your culture with other people.
- Identify your personality type and the personality types of the people whom you work with and consider how your similarities and differences can be assets at work.
- Find ways to take advantage of occupational and generational differences in the workplace.
- Treat all customers with respect; show special respect and appreciation for service and support workers.
- Focus on customer service strategies that result in high levels of patient satisfaction.
- Track patient satisfaction scores where you work and submit suggestions for improvement.
- Extend good customer service to the patients' family members, friends, and other visitors.
- Filter out the distractions around you in order to "be there" for your patients when they need you.
- Apply customer service standards when interacting with doctors, guests, and vendors.

Learning Activities

Using information from Chapter Five:
- Answer the Chapter Review Questions.
- Respond to the What If? Scenarios.
- Complete Chapter Five activities on the website.

Chapter Review Questions

Using information presented in Chapter Five, answer each of the following questions:

1. Give three examples of diversity in addition to age and gender.

2. Define the term *culture* and give three examples.

3. Define the terms *bias* and *disparities* and explain how bias can result in health care disparities for members of minority cultural groups.

4. Explain why health care workers need to be culturally competent.

5. Give two examples of generational differences and describe how they might affect someone's work.

6. List four types of health care customers.

7. Describe how hospitals are measuring and reporting patient satisfaction.

8. Describe five ways to provide good customer service for hospitalized patients and their visitors.

What If? Scenarios

Think about what you would do in the following situations and record your answers.

1. A hospitalized patient has a medical condition that you suffered yourself six months ago but the patient isn't aware of this. He asks if you have any idea what he can expect from his treatment plan.

2. You just moved from Maine to Southern California to start a new job. The majority of your clinic patients are immigrants from across the border. You've never been to Mexico yourself but you remember that your parents didn't like the Mexican family who lived next door when you were growing up in Maine.

3. You've been assigned to work on a project with four other members of your department. You've never worked with them before and it seems like you all have very different personalities.

4. Your supervisor is 45 years older than you. He constantly looks over your shoulder to make sure you're doing things correctly. If he would just give you the chance, you could computerize your office's financial records to make things quicker and easier to report.

5. Several people from your unit, including you, have been cross-trained to work in three different areas. Since all of you rotate on a weekly basis, none of you feel as if you really "belong" anywhere.

6. One of your patients scheduled for a procedure this morning has just informed you that she refuses to have the treatment.

7. It seems as if the patients from your hospital aren't as satisfied with the care they've received as compared with the patients from the two other hospitals in your town.

8. One of your patients seems depressed. She can't go home yet but her vital signs have improved considerably and she has regained her appetite.

9. A representative from a hospital supply company has arrived to meet with your manager. But your manager just got called into an emergency meeting and you have no idea when she'll be back.

10. Late this afternoon you took a phone call from a doctor in the sports medicine clinic who is upset about the delay in getting an x-ray report for a patient scheduled for surgery early tomorrow morning. The doctor got angry and called you unreliable even though you are just the receptionist who answers the phone.

PEARSON
myhealthprofessionskit™

Go to www.myhealthprofessionskit.com to access the Companion Website created for this textbook. Simply select "Basic Health Science" from the choice of disciplines. Find this book and log in using your username and password to access video scenarios, self-assessment quizzes, and more.

Professionalism and Your Personal Life

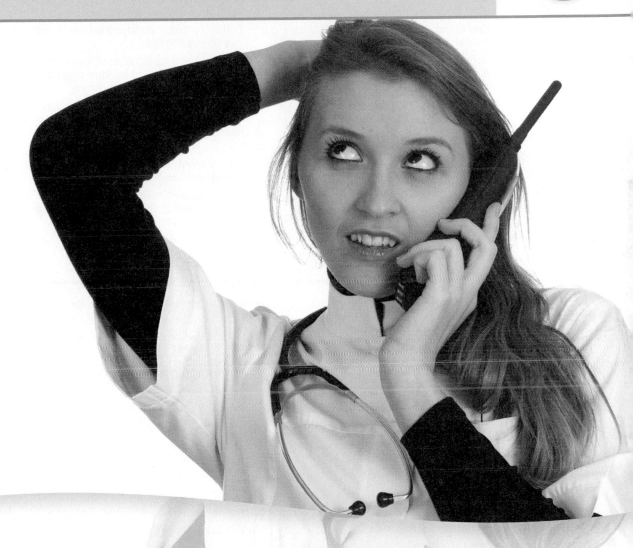

"We make a living by what we get, but we make a life by what we give."

Winston Churchill,
British Prime Minister, 1874–1965

CHAPTER OBJECTIVES

Having completed this chapter, you will be able to:

- Define *personal skills* and explain how they affect your success as a health care worker.
- Define *personal image* and describe how personal image affects patient care.
- List five appearance and grooming factors that result in a professional image.
- Discuss stereotypes and how they impact first impressions.
- List three examples of annoying and troublesome personal habits.
- Describe how grammar and vocabulary impact your professional image.
- Discuss the importance of maintaining professionalism after hours.

- Explain why health care employers are encouraging their employees to become healthier and give two examples.
- Define *personal management skills* and give three examples.
- Explain the importance of good time management skills and list three time management techniques.
- Explain the importance of good personal financial management skills and list three financial management techniques.
- Explain the importance of good stress management skills and list three stress management techniques.
- Define *adaptive skills* and explain why the ability to manage change is so important in health care today.

KEY TERMS

adaptive skills

body mass index (BMI)

dress code

grammar

health risk assessments

personal financial management

personal image

personal management skills

personal skills

posture

procrastinate

stress management

time management

well groomed

Personal Image

In previous chapters we've discussed how professionalism brings together who you are as a person and how you contribute those characteristics in the workplace. We've examined work ethic, character, morals, relationships, communication skills, diversity, and many other related topics. Now it's time to explore the connection between your personal life and your professional life.

You're just one person. It stands to reason that if your personal life is out of control, your professional life will suffer, too. When you have good **personal skills,** you're able to manage aspects of your life outside of work. This frees you up to concentrate on your job and your career. Of course, many of your personal skills transfer to the workplace and influence your reputation as a professional. This includes your personal image, personal health and wellness, and the ability to manage your time, finances, and stress and adapt to change. What does it take to have a well-orchestrated personal life that puts you on the right path to success in your career? Let's examine some personal skills and the impact they have on professionalism and success in the health care workplace.

One of the first things people notice about you is your **personal image**—the total impression you make on other people. Personal image includes your appearance, grooming, and **posture** (the position of the body or parts of the body); personal habits; and the **grammar** (system of word structures and arrangements) and language you use.

What kind of an impression do you make on people?

- Are you **well groomed** (clean and neat)?
- When you come to work, are you dressed properly to perform the duties of your job?
- Do your appearance and posture convey pride, competence, and professionalism?
- Do any personal habits detract from your image?
- How does your grammar or the language you use affect your personal image?

Appearance and Grooming

Your personal image is especially important in patient care. Patients need to have confidence in their caregivers. They want assurance that the people

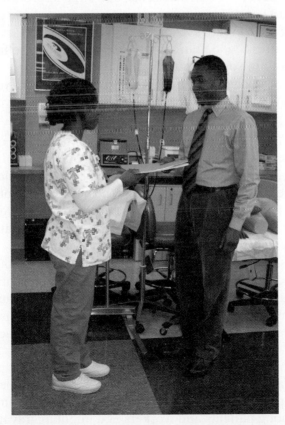

Figure 6-1 ■ Workers complying with standards for professional attire

caring for them are competent and professional. How would *you* feel if *your* caregiver had a ripped uniform, dirty shoes, oily hair, grimy fingernails, body odor, or bad breath? Would you wonder if that person's unprofessional appearance might also indicate a lack of pride or competence in his or her work?

Other people in addition to patients are affected by your personal appearance, too. Family members and friends who visit patients also need reassurance that their loved ones are being cared for by professionals. Vendors, guests, and other people who come into your workplace expect to see employees supporting a professional environment. Your coworkers and supervisor expect you to uphold the company's professional standards, too.

Then there's you. When you *look* good, you *feel* good. Setting high standards for your personal appearance not only conveys an image of professionalism to others, it also reinforces your pride and self-esteem. How can you expect others to view you as a professional if you don't look like or feel like a professional yourself?

Dress Codes

Most employers have a written **dress code** outlining appropriate and inappropriate attire. Dress code requirements may vary from department to department depending on the duties involved. For example, dietary workers would have a different dress code than secretaries. Be sure you're familiar with the dress code for your job and do your best to uphold it.

Consider the following as a general rule of thumb. If you don't wear a uniform, select clothing that's appropriate for the duties of your job.

- Your clothes should be clean, pressed, and fit properly. Avoid clothing that is wrinkled, frayed, too short, too tight, too baggy, or too revealing. Avoid clothes with wild colors and prints. Don't wear shirts or tops with messages printed on them unless approved by your employer.
- Avoid visible skin on your torso below the neckline of your shirt or top. This means no visible tummies, breasts, or back skin. Do not wear short shirts, short skirts, low-rise pants, or undergarments that are visible through your clothing.
- Your shoes should be clean, polished, and closed-toe. You must wear socks or stockings. No bare feet, slippers, flip-flops, or open-toe shoes.
- Keep makeup, jewelry, and other accessories to a minimum and in good taste. In some health care professions such as dental assisting, no jewelry is allowed. Avoid brightly polished fingernails and acrylic, artificial nails.
- Long hair should be pulled back and secured to avoid sanitary or safety problems. Facial hair should be groomed and neatly styled.
- Never wear perfume, aftershave, or scented lotions. Aromas may not be welcome among patients and workers and might aggravate breathing difficulties.

- Poor posture can undermine a professional image. Sit up straight, stand erect, and don't slouch.
- Wear your employee identification badge as prescribed in your company's dress code.
- Avoid non-traditional hairstyles and colors, cover up tattoos, and remove facial piercings.

Remember, you don't come to work to set new fashion trends or win a beauty contest. Your clothing and accessories should support getting your work done efficiently and safely while instilling a feeling of confidence among those you serve.

- Save your evening wear, party attire, sportswear, and the latest fashions for after hours.
- Shorts, capris, leggings, cropped pants, tight pants, tank tops, bare back tops, miniskirts, midriff tops, athletic attire, sweatshirts, sweatpants, T-shirts, painter pants, bib overalls, spaghetti strap dresses, reflective clothing, see-through fabrics, low or revealing necklines, spandex tops and pants, untucked shirttails, and visible undergarments are never acceptable.
- On "casual days," remember that you're still in the workplace. If your job involves contact with patients and other customers, avoid wearing blue jeans, T-shirts, or other questionable attire even on casual days.

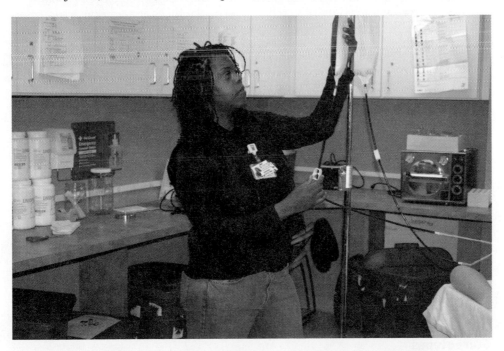

Figure 6-2 ■ Worker in denim jeans dressed unprofessionally

- Many health care employers ban any type of clothing made of denim including scrubs, skirts, shirts, pants, dresses, and jeans regardless of the color.
- Sunglasses should not be worn unless for medical reasons. The use of head coverings is limited to religious customs or job-specific regulations.

Keep in mind that what constitutes a professional image to one person might be quite different from that which constitutes a professional image to another person. In other words, professional image "is in the eye of the beholder." Such differences often relate to the age and generation of the beholder. Appearance factors that may seem appropriate for your age group may be disturbing to other people, especially those older than you. This includes such things as facial piercings, non-traditional hairstyles and colors, and tattoos.

CONSIDER THIS

CHANGES IN DRESS CODES OVER TIME

Many years ago, female nurses had to wear white, starched, uniform dresses and caps on their heads. Have you seen such attire in *any* hospital in recent years? Facial hair on men used to be highly discouraged. Now, as long as facial hair is groomed, it's rarely an issue. Years ago, women were expected to wear skirts at work because pants were considered unprofessional. Today, women wearing pants at work is the norm. In the not-so-distant past, only surgery employees could wear scrubs. Today, the majority of caregivers wear scrubs. Standardizing scrub colors and styles helps patients and other people differentiate among registered nurses, licensed practical nurses, nurse aids, support staff, technologists, and other types of health care workers.

Based on history, dress codes of tomorrow may be less rigid than those of today. As younger generations enter the workforce in large numbers, dress code requirements may change but health care companies tend to be conservative and it can take a long time for dress codes to evolve. Depending on where you work and what job you have, dress code requirements may limit opportunities to express your individuality. You may have to dress like everyone else in your department, practice, or office. You may be subject to a dress code that was developed by people significantly older than you. Adherence to dress code policies is a requirement of your job. Always think twice about attire, accessories, or other aspects of personal appearance that might make someone else feel uncomfortable or question your professionalism or competence. When you're at work, it's all about the patient and other customers—not you.

Stereotypes

Stereotyping can affect your personal image at work. Stereotypes are often based on personal appearance. When older people, for example, see members of the younger generation with facial piercings, tattoos, and unusual hairstyles, they form first impressions based on their stereotypes. First impressions aren't usually accurate but they still occur. If someone negatively stereotypes you, once they get to know you and observe your behavior, their impression may improve over time. In the meantime, however, some patients may ask to have a "different" health care worker take care of them, wanting someone who better fits their stereotype of a professional-looking person. Young people may also form first impressions of older people, again based on stereotypes and inaccurate judgments. Stereotyping is a fact of life but if you're aware of it, you can counteract its negative impact. Try to avoid stereotyping and judging other people yourself. Give everyone you meet the benefit of the doubt and don't rely on first impressions.

When discussing stereotyping, the topic of weight needs to be addressed briefly. Although it's a sensitive issue, people who are extremely overweight may notice an adverse reaction when seeking employment. Although we would like to believe that body weight is not a factor in employment decisions, it sometimes happens. Overweight people may be stereotyped as lazy and unable to muster self-discipline. Yet in reality, one's weight may have no bearing on productivity and self-control.

The issue of limited space may come into play. A manager may say, "We can't consider him for this job because the space he would have to work in is too cramped and confining for him to function properly." In surgery, there may be concerns about an obese nurse or surgical technologist contaminating a sterile field when working in a cramped environment. In radiology, equipment controls may be housed in cubicles too confining for a large person. In jobs requiring heavy lifting or frequent physical activity, employers may feel that such activities could jeopardize the health and safety of an overweight worker.

Although it's unfortunate that a person's body weight could have a negative impact on his or her career, it is a fact of life. If you are seriously overweight and wish to do something about it, work closely with your family physician to plan a safe and healthy course of action. If you're content with your weight, or for medical reasons are unable to reduce your weight, be on the lookout for employment opportunities in which weight is not a factor. Weight and other topics related to personal health and wellness will be discussed later in this chapter.

Personal Habits

Your habits are also part of your personal image and they can sometimes be annoying or troublesome to those around you. Here are some suggestions:

- Don't wear noisy shoes or jewelry that jangles.
- Don't chew gum, pop your knuckles, or bite your fingernails.
- Don't play jokes and childish pranks on coworkers.
- Avoid making a mess when eating or drinking in your work area.

- If you have a hearing loss, get fitted for hearing aids; asking people to repeat things can become annoying.
- Don't play music loud enough for other people around you to hear it.
- Don't forward chain e-mail messages to coworkers.
- Don't use business computers for personal purposes.
- Don't use personal cell phones or send text messages during work hours.
- Don't congregate with coworkers in patient or visitor areas before or after your shift.

There are lots of other do's and don'ts, many of which relate to etiquette and manners. Always think about how your actions might affect other people.

Most health care companies are smoke-free. If employees must smoke, they're directed to designated "smoking huts" or they stand outside the building, huddled together on public sidewalks. As you might imagine, this doesn't present a very professional image to the public. Some health care employers have a total campus-wide ban on smoking and won't allow employees on-site if their clothing smells like smoke. If you must smoke:

- Make sure you're familiar with your company's smoking policies.
- Confine smoking to designated areas to protect others from secondhand smoke.
- Avoid taking too many smoking breaks or breaks that last too long.

Don't appear for work smelling of cigarette, cigar, or pipe smoke. Many people are allergic to smoke. Patients are ill and the smell of smoke can be detrimental to their comfort.

An increasing number of health care employers require job applicants to undergo drug/nicotine screens and they won't hire people who smoke. Some employers charge higher premiums on health insurance benefits for employees who smoke. Just as obesity may have an adverse affect on job opportunities, so may smoking. It's hard to maintain your professional image when engulfed in a cloud of smoke or wearing clothing that reeks of cigarettes, cigars, or pipes. Many employers offer free smoking cessation classes for their employees. If you smoke and wish to quit, join a support group and get your doctor's advice on how to proceed.

Language and Grammar

Another habit that may annoy people at work is the language you use. Don't refer to people has *honey, sweetie,* or *dear.* Adult males are *men,* not *boys* or *guys.* Adult females are *women,* not *girls* or *gals.* Don't assume that an older female is a *Mrs.* It's best to refer to females as *Miss* or *Ms.*

Some language is totally unacceptable in the workplace, including obscene, cursing, and vulgar language; sexually explicit or risqué comments; and terms that demean members of any racial, cultural, or ethnic group. "Street language" that might be acceptable after hours with your family or friends may be viewed as inappropriate by coworkers, patients, or visitors.

Words such as *fart*, *suck*, *pissed off*, and *ass* are becoming common in public but are still considered inappropriate in the workplace.

Telling jokes in poor taste and making "off-color" remarks is not a good idea, even during breaks. Remember the prior discussion about sexual harassment and creating an uncomfortable work environment for others? Even if you mean no harm, someone else's perception might be different than yours. Always be respectful of other people's points of view and avoid using language they might find offensive.

Grammar also plays a role in your personal and professional image. Poor grammar signals a lack of education and refinement. It's not uncommon for people to mismatch the subject and verb in a sentence. Here are some examples:

- "We was there" should be "We *were* there."
- "I seen you do that" should be "I *saw* you do that."
- "Me and him" should be "he and I."
- "She don't know" should be "She *doesn't* know."
- "Her and I" should be "she and I."

Poor grammar is learned and then reinforced by the people with whom you associate. Poor grammar starts with your family as a child and expands to your friends and coworkers. Contemporary music, advertisements, and the media also reinforce poor grammar (such as the song lyric, "It don't matter to me"). If the people who are close to you use incorrect grammar, it's likely you will, too, without even realizing it. Just being aware of the need for good grammar might help. If your grammar is weak, work toward improving it. You might be surprised how much it can affect your personal and professional image.

Remember the old saying, "You only get one chance to make a good first impression"? In health care, *every* impression you make is important. As discussed previously, to patients and other customers, *you* are the company you work for. If you appear less than professional, so might your company. Put together a total personal package that portrays a professional image. It's a big part of your job and it can make or break your reputation as a professional.

Maintaining Professionalism After Hours

At first glance you might not realize it, but even when you're away from work your behavior can affect your professional image. For example, how do you answer your telephone? What impression does your ring tone make on people who hear it? What kind of impression does your recorded telephone message make on people who call you? Don't assume that every caller is a friend, family member, or stranger trying to sell you something. What if your supervisor calls or a potential employer? Your telephone is an extension of your personal image so think about who might be calling you and the impression you want to make.

Your relationships at work and outside of work can also have a positive or negative effect on your personal and professional image. The types of people with whom you associate are a reflection of your personal values and who you are as a person. What effect do the people with whom *you* associate have on your reputation?

It's a small world. You never know when you might run into your supervisor, a coworker, or someone who knows someone you know after hours. "So what?" you might ask. "If I'm not at work, what difference does it make? What I do on my own time is no one's business." Although it's true that you are "off the clock," what you do after hours can make a huge difference. Your reputation goes with you *everyplace* you go. You never know who might be sitting across the room from you in a restaurant, bar, or some other public place. If you've had a few drinks and your voice gets loud, and you spread gossip, reveal confidential information, or criticize your employer in public, you could be subject to serious problems at work. If you call in sick when you really aren't and then go out in public, you never know whom you might run into. If someone sees you and word gets back to your supervisor, you wouldn't be the first person to get fired from a job under circumstances like these. If you're arrested and spend the night in jail, don't be surprised if your employer finds out.

If your work group, department, or company has a special event after hours, the standards that govern acceptable behavior at work apply during those events, too. Always conduct yourself in a professional manner. Don't drink too much, engage in wild behavior, and then regret it the next day. It's hard to reestablish trust, respect, and your professional reputation after making some poor decisions the night before. Be very careful about what you post on Facebook, Twitter, and other Internet social networking sites and blogs. Sharing personal photographs and private information, posting complaints and gossip about coworkers and your employer, and making even casual comments about patients are easy ways to ruin your reputation and lead to corrective action or dismissal from your job.

Give serious thought to the pros and cons of dating someone you work with before you decide to do it. How might having a personal relationship outside of work affect both of you at work? What might happen if the relationship ends? Could the other person end up being your supervisor someday or your subordinate? What issues related to sexual harassment might arise? If you're dating your supervisor and things go wrong, you may have to change jobs. If you "mix business with pleasure" with people who report to you, you may have difficulty supervising them later on. It's best to avoid these kinds of social relationships because they often lead to trouble.

The point of this discussion is to remember that you are just one person. You aren't one person at work and a different person after work, so do your best to maintain a positive image after hours, too. It is okay to "let your hair down" and have a good time but don't let your guard down as well. Always think before you act.

RECENT DEVELOPMENTS

SOCIAL NETWORKING SITES AND YOUR JOB

Any content that you post on the Internet or that other people post about you is public information that can affect your professional reputation. Employers now visit social networking sites and review blogs to track down personal information about job applicants and current employees. New policies now lead to corrective action or dismissal when employees display an unprofessional image online. This might not seem fair since your Facebook page or blog, for example, is your own private business. But employers see things differently. Remember the statement, "*You* are the company you work for."

If your employer spots photographs of you naked, drunk, engaged in illegal activities, or doing anything else they believe might undermine the reputation of the company, they may decide you are no longer a good fit for the organization. Don't post anything online that might cause embarrassment or worse at work.

Personal Health and Wellness

Health care is one of most physically demanding, emotionally draining, and stressful industries in which to work. Meeting the needs of patients, operating hightech equipment, dealing with lean staffing, adhering to tight schedules, and handling life-and-death situations on a daily basis can result in high levels of stress. Lifting patients and heavy objects can cause back injuries, and employees can catch infectious diseases from patients, visitors, and guests. So it's important to pay attention to your own health and wellness while caring for other people. Watch for signs of stress, practice safe lifting techniques, ensure your vaccinations are up-to-date, and use standard precautions to guard against infectious disease.

Health care costs are continuing to rise in the United States and rising costs create financial difficulties for employers who provide health insurance for their employees. As the cost of health care increases, employers must cover the extra expense themselves, charge employees more for their coverage, or reduce the health care benefits their employees receive. When you stop and think about it, health care companies are employers, too. They must figure out how to handle the rising cost of health insurance for their employees.

These financial pressures have resulted in a variety of programs to encourage employees to become healthier. In some companies, employees get a discount on their health insurance when they meet certain health indicators. In other companies, employees are charged higher rates for their health insurance when they fail to meet certain health indicators. Either way you look at it, these financial incentives are generating visible improvements in the way health care workers manage their own health.

THINK ABOUT IT

CAREGIVERS AS ROLE MODELS

Research shows that patients who smoke are less likely to stop smoking if their caregivers smoke themselves. Although doctors, nurses, and respiratory therapists encourage their patients to refrain from smoking, their efforts are less successful when they don't practice what they preach themselves. Patients view their caregivers as educators and trusted role models. When their caregivers continue to smoke despite the overwhelming evidence that smoking is hazardous to their health, then patients are less likely to follow the advice given by their caregivers. One of the strategies, therefore, to reduce smoking among the general public is to reduce smoking among health care workers.

Health care companies want their employees to set a good example for patients and the community when it comes to health and wellness. They're offering voluntary "wellness tracks" that include the following:

- **Health risk assessments** These are questionnaires that identify which health issues you need to focus on based on your medical history and lifestyle.
- Health screenings that measure **body mass index (BMI)** (measure of body fat based on height and weight for adult men and women), blood pressure, blood glucose, and cholesterol

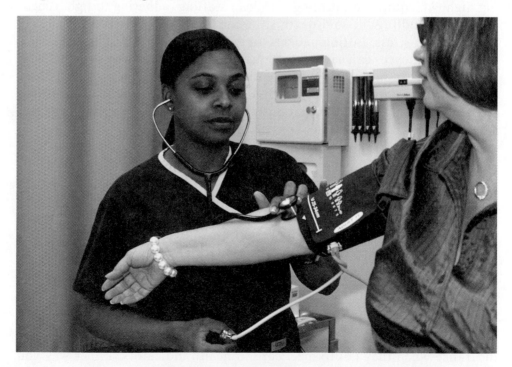

Figure 6-3 ■ Worker undergoing a wellness blood pressure check

CASE STUDY

It's been several months since Carla started working with her new team and she's realized that things have really changed with her job. As part of her duties as team leader for the Patient Experience sub-committee, she's been visiting several out-of-town clinics known for their outstanding customer service and high patient satisfaction scores. She's read dozens of articles and reports about customer service in 5-star restaurants and hotels and thought about how their approaches might apply in health care. She's convened two focus groups of patients to ask them what they feel is important when receiving clinic-based services. She's learning far more than she ever expected in such a short period of time. And she's really glad that she still gets to work as a medical assistant about 20 hours a week to maintain her skills and contact with patients.

Carla's role has changed dramatically. She's out in front now, meeting with doctors, conversing with patients, negotiating with vendors, and giving reports at staff meetings. Her hard work has certainly paid off but now she's beginning to wonder if her personal image needs some sprucing up. She isn't used to giving presentations and participating in high-level meetings but she knows she has to look the part. She's beginning to wonder if she should lose some weight, get in better shape, and buy some clothes other than scrubs.

What should Carla do, if anything, to make sure that her appearance and her overall personal image support the success she's experienced in her new role? What, if anything, would you do if you were in Carla's place?

- Exercise, nutrition, weight loss, smoking cessation, and stress **management** classes (the ability to deal with stress and overcome stressful situations)
- Coaching and support provided by wellness counselors

Employers are offering healthier food in their cafeterias and vending machines, setting aside bicycle and walking paths on their campuses, planting gardens to provide fresh produce, and offering employee discounts on memberships at local fitness clubs. All of this is good news for health care workers who recognize the connection between a healthy personal life and a healthy professional live.

Personal Management Skills

Personal management skills (the ability to manage time, personal finances, stress, and change) help you keep your personal life in order and support your success at work. Attendance and punctuality are good examples of how your personal life can affect your job. After all, does it really matter how professional you look or how competent you are if you can't get to work on time and be there when you're supposed to be? Your ability to show up for work on a daily basis and keep your appointments is one important aspect of your job.

If you have trouble managing your time, handling your finances, dealing with stress, or adapting to change, your personal life could have a negative impact on your job and your career. Let's take a closer look.

Time Management

When it seems as if there are never enough hours in the day to get everything done that needs to get done, **time management** skills (the ability to organize and allocate one's time to increase productivity) can be a big help. Here are some suggestions to help you balance work, family, and the many other priorities in your life:

- Use an electronic or pocket-sized calendar to record your work schedule, classes, appointments, and so on. Refer to your calendar every day and think about what's coming up tomorrow so you can be prepared.
- Don't schedule things too closely together, allow extra time for travel, and have contingency plans for unexpected complications.
- Make lists of things that need to get done. If you become overwhelmed, decide which are the most important and which you can let go.
- Eliminate activities that waste time and learn to say "no" when you're overbooked.
- Don't **procrastinate** (to postpone or delay taking action). Letting things build up is a sure way to become overwhelmed and disorganized.

Identify your priorities and allocate your time accordingly. You can't create more hours in the day but you can seize control of the time you have. After all, time is one of your most precious and most limited commodities. Learning how to manage it appropriately can have a positive impact on your personal and professional life.

Personal Financial Management

How well you manage another precious and limited commodity—your personal finances—also can have a big impact your personal and professional life. Effective **personal financial management** skills (the ability to make sound decisions about personal finances) can help you pay your bills on time and avoid financial problems that could cause embarrassment at work. Here are some suggestions to help you live within your means and avoid wasting money:

- Develop a budget, monitor your expenses, and know where your money is going. Keep your checking and savings accounts balanced. Match up paydays with the dates you pay your bills to avoid getting charged late fees.
- Read the fine print on loan and credit card applications. Avoid the high cost of doing business with companies that offer check-cashing services, payday loans, rent-to-own furniture, and income tax–refund anticipation loans.

- Limit credit card use to emergency situations or to make purchases that you already have the cash to cover. Aim for a zero balance on credit cards to avoid paying high interest fees.
- Have a savings plan and stick with it. Put some money away for emergencies and other unexpected expenses. Start saving now for retirement. You'll be surprised how quickly small investments can grow.
- Think twice before loaning someone money or cosigning on a loan. If you must loan money, use a written agreement detailing plans for repayment.
- Ask if liability insurance is recommended for people in your profession. This is especially important for some types of licensed professionals.

Managing personal finances can be quite a challenge in today's world. Establish priorities for how you want to allocate your resources and make your financial decisions accordingly.

Stress Management

As mentioned previously, health care jobs are among the most stress-producing occupations in the nation. Stress can affect your physical health as well as your mental and emotional health. Many physicians and researchers are convinced that stress is a contributing factor to several different diseases and abnormalities. Stress can make you sick and cause symptoms such as headaches, fatigue, sleep problems, diarrhea, indigestion, ulcers, hypertension, dizziness, hives, grinding teeth, skin disorders, and stuttering. Stress has been linked with heart attacks, high blood pressure, alcoholism, depression, and drug abuse.

People with Type A personalities are among the most susceptible to stress-related disorders. They are highly competitive, impatient, high achievers with strong perfectionist tendencies. They often rush from place to place, work long hours, have an intense drive to get things done, become frustrated easily, and have trouble relaxing. When Type A personalities have a lifestyle that includes smoking, drinking, a poor diet, a lack of exercise, and obesity, they become targets for stress-related illness. If you're a Type A personality yourself, or if the stress you experience tends to affect your health in any way, don't wait until it's too late. Watch for the warning signs and seek help to deal with it.

Effective stress management skills can be quite valuable in your personal life and at work. Managing stress is a key factor in your image as a professional. If you blow up, melt down, or run for the door at the first sign of stress, you may be letting down your coworkers and patients. Your ability to perform the duties of your job may be affected and your personal health and wellness may suffer. Good stress management techniques can help you keep everything in balance and add more enjoyment to your life. Here are some suggestions:

- Become aware of when, how, and why stress is affecting you; identify where the stress is coming from; and seek ways to reduce or eliminate the stress.
- Identify someone you can talk with—a person who can relate to what you're experiencing and help you think through it.

- Try to keep work-related stress from affecting your personal life and try to keep stress in your personal life from affecting your job and your work. This is easier said than done.
- Maintain a healthy balance among work, recreation, and rest. Use your vacation time wisely. Learn to relax and schedule time for hobbies, sports, and other personal interests. Get plenty of sleep and exercise and eat properly.
- Use your conflict resolution skills when necessary and avoid keeping negative feelings bottled up inside you.

An important part of managing stress is being well adjusted and finding happiness in life. Professionals have a positive self-image. They have high levels of self-esteem and self-respect and they know they are worthy individuals. Let's face it—it's difficult for others to have confidence in you if you don't have confidence in yourself. These suggestions can help you build confidence:

- Look for the good in yourself, know your limits, and work within them.
- Be patient with yourself and with others. Avoid being a perfectionist— no one is perfect. Setting unrealistic goals is counterproductive and leads to disappointment, low self-esteem, and unnecessary stress.
- Set high but realistic standards for yourself and feel good about your accomplishments.

Learn to manage your stress and find ways to achieve happiness at work and at home. Making the most of change is a good place to start.

Managing Change

In today's health care workplace, one of the most important personal management skills is the ability to adjust to change. Just when you think everything is arranged as it should be, something changes. You might acquire extra job duties, undergo cross-training, or be assigned to work in a different location. Your work schedule might get altered, your company might merge with another company, or your supervisor might change. At the same time you're affected by changes at work, you're probably facing changes in your personal life, too. Family responsibilities, relationships with friends, and pressures involving finances, housing, and personal health can all cause many changes over the course of your life.

It's almost impossible to avoid change. If you're the type of person who resists change, you're going to face some difficult struggles working in health care. However, if you have effective **adaptive skills** (the ability to adjust to change), you'll be well prepared for the many changes that life will throw your way.

Years ago, health care workers were encouraged to *cope* with change. When the pace of change increased, people were encouraged to *manage* change. Now that change is occurring so rapidly, health care workers must *embrace* change and even *lead* change from time to time.

Change can be a positive influence in your life if you learn to accept it and let it open new doors for you. Having your job redesigned, for example, can be pretty scary. You might have to learn some new skills and take on new responsibilities but the more new challenges you face, the more you will grow. The more you grow, the better your chances for advancement. View change as positive and learn to make it work *for* you instead of *against* you. After all, do you really want your personal life and your career to be exactly the same five years from now as they are today?

For More Information

Body Mass Index
National Heart, Lung and Blood Institute
U.S. Department of Health and Human Services
www.nhlbisupport.com/bmi/
301-592-8573

Time Management Strategies and Techniques
For individuals, managers, and students
Resources, tips, and tools
www.timemanagement.com

Stress Management
MedLine Plus
U.S. National Library of Medicine and The National Institutes of Health
www.nlm.nih.gov/medlineplus

Personal Financial Management
Kiplinger
www.kiplinger.com

Health Risk Assessments
Free Heart Attack Risk Assessment
American Heart Association
http://www.heart.org/HEARTORG/ Conditions/HeartAttack/ HeartAttackToolsResources/ Heart-Attack-Risk-Assessment_ UCM_303944_Article.jsp
800-242-8721

REALITY CHECK

It's time to get real and take a close look at the personal image that you portray. Do your appearance, habits, language, and grammar lead people to view you as a professional? Or would patients, coworkers, and doctors question your competence because of your attire or the condition of the clothes you wear? Do you take into account how elderly people might react to your appearance? Or is your unsettling image leading patients to ask for someone different to take care of them? Are you careful about what you say at work and how you say it? Or is using street language offending people and damaging your reputation?

You might be amazed at how some people show up for work. They look like they just rolled out of bed or never went to bed. It's obvious they either don't care what they look like or they don't have a clue how people are expected to dress in a business environment. Once you've made a negative impression, it will be difficult to overcome people's opinions of you. Bare skin, visible undergarments, and spandex clothes could be enough to shock your supervisor into putting you on corrective action and sending you home without pay. If any of this describes you, it's time to clean up your act and your appearance.

Key Points

- Do your best to keep your personal life in balance so that personal problems don't have a negative impact on your professional reputation.
- Adhere to dress code policies to portray a positive personal image.
- Choose clothing and accessories that allow you to perform your work efficiently and safely.
- Avoid stereotyping other people and forming inaccurate first impressions.
- Avoid personal habits that annoy other people.
- Use proper language and grammar and avoid street language at work.
- Don't let your guard down after hours.
- Think twice before dating a coworker or your supervisor.
- Take advantage of health risk assessments and address medical conditions uncovered.
- Use good time management skills and don't procrastinate.
- Keep your personal finances in order and live within your means.
- Identify the sources of your stress and take steps to reduce or eliminate them.
- Sharpen your adaptive skills and be open to opportunities that come with change.

Learning Activities

Using information from Chapter Six:
- Answer the Chapter Review Questions.
- Respond to the What If? Scenarios.
- Complete Chapter Six activities on the website.

Chapter Review Questions

Using information presented in Chapter Six, answer each of the following questions:
1. Define *personal skills* and explain how they affect your success as a health care worker.

2. Define *personal image* and describe how personal image affects patient care.

3. List five appearance and grooming factors that result in a professional image.

4. Discuss stereotypes and how they impact first impressions.

5. List three examples of annoying and troublesome personal habits.

6. Describe how grammar and vocabulary impact your professional image.

7. Discuss the importance of maintaining professionalism after hours.

8. Explain why health care employers are encouraging their employees to become healthier and give two examples.

9. Define *personal management skills* and give three examples.

10. Explain the importance of good time management skills and list three time management techniques.

11. Explain the importance of good personal financial management skills and list three financial management techniques.

12. Explain the importance of good stress management skills and list three stress management techniques.

13. Define *adaptive skills* and explain why the ability to manage change is so important in health care today.

What If? Scenarios

Think about what you would do in the following situations and record your answers.

1. Your company's dress code allows denim jeans and T-shirts on Fridays for "casual day." Because you've been cross-trained to fill in for the customer service department when it is shorthanded, it's possible you could be asked to work at the information desk in the main lobby with little or no notice.

2. You've spent six months working out at a fitness center and look really good in tight blouses and short skirts. Hopefully, the cute guy who started working in medical records last week will notice you and ask you out.

3. Some of the employees with whom you eat lunch use crude language and at times it can be overheard by other people in your company's cafeteria.

4. The only free time you have to jog on a regular basis is during your lunch break. Your break is long enough to get some good exercise, but you don't have time to take a shower before resuming work.

5. You and a group of coworkers decide to start meeting at a popular bar on Saturday nights to "let your hair down" and have a good time. On the very first night, one person in your group drinks too much and ends up in a fistfight with a stranger seated at the next table. You overhear the bartender calling the police.

6. It seems there are never enough hours in the day for you to get everything done that you want to do. You work full time, participate in two bowling leagues, transport your children to sporting events, volunteer at a local golf course, play basketball with your friends on Saturday afternoon, and take two courses each semester toward the degree you've been working on. Last week, you were late for work twice, called in sick the day your son's school was closed because of the weather, and had to cancel a dentist appointment at the last minute. You know your job is important but so are your family, friends, and other activities.

7. You just received a pay raise, giving you an extra $25 in each paycheck. Then the telephone rang and you found out you qualified for a new credit card that you hadn't even applied for. With your pay raise and a $5,000 credit limit, you've got the money you need to buy that new flat screen television your children have been begging you for.

8. For the past month, you've been having headaches and difficulty sleeping at night. You're less patient with your children and have yelled at them several times. Even though you've been eating more than usual, you seem to have very little energy and can't keep up with physical activities. Yesterday, when your supervisor asked if you could work overtime, you blew up and yelled, "Are you kidding me? Why can't somebody else do it? Why does it always have to be me?"

9. You just found out that your health insurance premium at work is going up $50 a month. If you fill out a health risk assessment, undergo a physical exam, and fall within the healthy range for indicators such as blood pressure and body mass index, you can reduce your cost by $25 a month.

10. Someone that you thought was your friend just posted embarrassing photographs of you taken at a party last weekend without your permission. Within minutes, several friends texted you to make sure you knew the photos were on the Internet. Now you're afraid your boss will find out.

PEARSON
myhealthprofessionskit™

Go to www.myhealthprofessionskit.com to access the Companion Website created for this textbook. Simply select "Basic Health Science" from the choice of disciplines. Find this book and log in using your username and password to access video scenarios, self-assessment quizzes, and more.

7

The Practicum Experience

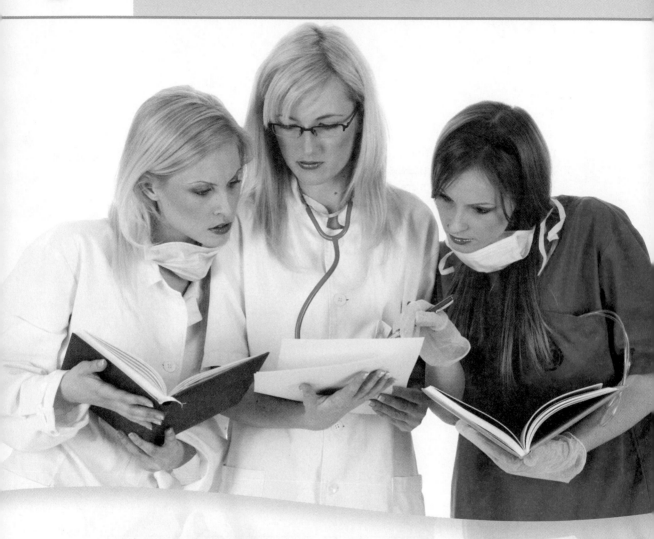

"My interest is in the future because I am going to spend the rest of my life there."

Charles F. Kettering,
Inventor and engineer, 1876–1958

CHAPTER OBJECTIVES

Having completed this chapter, you will be able to:

- Identify the purpose of a practicum.
- List three benefits of a practicum experience.
- Describe three ways to prepare for a practicum.
- Discuss four examples of proper behavior while on a practicum.
- Describe three ways to ensure success during a practicum.
- Explain the importance of patient confidentiality during a practicum.

- Discuss the value of keeping a journal during a practicum.
- Explain the importance of putting the practicum site first.
- Describe the connection between a practicum and employment after graduation.
- Identify four general policies, procedures, and issues related to a successful practicum experience.
- Define the term *protocol*.

KEY TERMS

journal	office politics	profane	samples room
observations	penmanship	protocol	

The Purpose of a Practicum

A practicum is a real-life learning experience obtained through working on-site in a health care facility while enrolled as a student. Educational programs use different terms for the practicum experience, such as *clinicals, externship, internship, hands-on experience,* and so forth, but these terms all mean basically the same thing. Whether you're in medical assisting, surgical technology, radiography, medical technology, or another type of health care educational program, there's a good chance you'll be doing a practicum learning experience before you graduate. Some programs begin the practicum experience early in the curriculum, integrating classroom instruction with hands-on experience. Other programs complete classroom instruction first and schedule the practicum at the end of the program just before graduation.

The Benefits of a Practicum Experience

You may be thinking, "Should I worry about my practicum? Isn't it just another assignment to complete before I can graduate?" In reality, your practicum is much more than just another assignment. In fact, it's probably *the* most important part of your education. Your practicum is an opportunity to apply the knowledge and skills you've acquired during the classroom (or online) portion of your training in an actual health care setting while still a student. If you perform well, your practicum could also result in an employment recommendation or a job offer when you graduate.

Student Versus Employee

Practicum experiences vary in length, depending on the discipline you're studying and the program you're enrolled in. Some practicums will be relatively short, lasting just a few weeks or months. Other practicums will extend over several months or even a year or more. Since educational accreditation requirements usually don't allow students to be paid during their practicum, at times you may feel like you are giving away free labor. Keep one very important fact in mind—you are there as a *student* to learn and to hone your knowledge and skills. Even though the site supervisor will assign your work hours, break times, duties, and responsibilities, you are *not* there as an employee. There's a big difference between being on-site as a student and working there as an employee. You need to keep these differences in mind as you progress through the experience.

Participating in a practicum is a privilege. Whether your practicum is in a hospital, outpatient clinic, physician practice, surgery or imaging center, or clinical lab, you are a guest in the facility. The site supervisor has the right to terminate your practicum at any point in time if he or she believes that your appearance, attitude, or performance negatively affects the site's patients, visitors, physicians, or employees. So you must prove yourself in the early stages of your practicum to convince the site supervisor that you are prepared and personally committed to performing well. It's time to apply everything you've learned and begin establishing your own reputation as a health care professional.

Identifying Preferences

Another benefit of your practicum is having the opportunity to decide what types of patients you'd like to work with after you graduate. It's not unusual to hear students say they want to work in pediatrics (peds). Working with pediatric patients can be highly rewarding but it takes a certain type of person to do this. Sometimes students have an unrealistic image of what it takes to work with children. They imagine themselves holding and cuddling newborns and small children. They don't always think about the children being sick and their parents being anxious and upset. Experience shows that about half of the students who say they want to work in peds change their minds after a pediatric practicum. Radiography students who think they want to specialize in neuro procedures or surgical technology students who think they want to scrub in on cardiovascular cases may change their minds after working with these types of patients during their practicum.

The same may be true for different employment locations. Pharmacy technician students may think that working in a hospital pharmacy would be their first choice after graduation, and physical therapy assistants may set their sights on outpatient rehabilitation centers. After their practicums, the pharmacy techs might decide on retail pharmacies and the physical therapy assistants might seek jobs in acute care hospitals. There's nothing like being there to know for sure where you'd like to work and the types of patients and procedures you'd like to be involved with. Your practicum can help you make those decisions before you apply for jobs and accept an offer.

CONSIDER THIS

SITE ORIENTATION

Health care companies are highly focused on customer service and patient satisfaction. Protecting their reputations in order to remain competitive is a high priority. Even though you'll be a student in your practicum site, you might be issued a site ID badge to wear while you're there. The site's patients, visitors, and guests may assume that you are part of the company. Your appearance, attitude, and behavior will affect the site's reputation so it's important to be familiar with their mission, vision, and values.

Expect to participate in a site-specific orientation when you start your practicum. This orientation may be short, such as conversation with your site supervisor, or it might involve attending a full-day orientation session with some of the site's employees who are starting their new jobs. Pay attention and do your best to help the site maintain and enhance its reputation in the community.

Performance Evaluation

Your performance during your practicum will be evaluated based on criteria established by your educational program. You will likely receive a grade based on your attendance, attitude, appearance, and overall performance so it's important to do your best. The employees who work at the site know that you're a student. They expect you to be a little bit nervous at first and won't hold you accountable for knowing everything when you start. But if it's clear that you haven't been well trained before starting your practicum, your deficiencies will become apparent pretty quickly. Feel free to ask questions and show an interest in what goes on at the site but don't ask the same question repeatedly. Remember the answer and jot it down on a small, pocket notepad.

Picture a practicum site with two students. One student is always visible, asking questions, stepping in to help, and taking notes. The other student is usually off someplace, socializing or taking a smoke break. She rarely asks questions, doesn't show much initiative, and always has some reason why she has to leave early every week. It should be obvious which student will earn the higher grade. But what neither student knows is there's going to be a position opening up about the same time the practicum ends and the students graduate. In situations such as this, the practicum wasn't just another assignment but actually a multi-week job interview.

Recent Developments

GAINING CLEARANCE

Health care companies are becoming more selective with the students they accept for practicum experience as a result of growing concerns about workplace theft and violence, sexual harassment, breach of patient confidentiality, and unauthorized sharing of private business information. As a result, the requirements that students must meet to gain clearance for a practicum experience are becoming increasingly restrictive.

To be cleared for a practicum, expect to undergo a criminal history background check, drug test, and physical exam. If you anticipate problems passing a background check or drug screen, discuss the situation with your instructor as soon as possible. You also may need to prove that you'll be covered by personal health insurance during the practicum period.

With respect to vaccinations, you'll either have to submit documentation from your personal physician that you've had the vaccinations or before starting your practicum you'll need to receive the vaccinations, which include mumps, rubella, varicella, measles, tetanus, diphtheria, and pertussis. Many sites also require students to have an annual flu shot. Depending on your program and the types of patients you'll be working with, you may also need the Hepatitis B vaccination (or be required to sign a waiver form) and be fit tested for an N95 respirator. If your practicum is lengthy, expect to undergo an annual TB test.

Preparing for Your Practicum

Depending on your educational program, you may be assigned to a practicum site or you may have some choices. If you have choices, there are some important things to consider before making your decision.

Don't choose a practicum site where you or your family members are patients. It's best to choose a location where you can be viewed solely as a student. It's also preferable to choose a site where you don't know the patients. Having personal relationships with patients at your practicum site can create issues with privacy and confidentiality.

Pre-Practicum Observations and Research

Some educational programs schedule on-site **observations** for students to visit potential sites before selecting or being assigned to a practicum location. Take advantage of this opportunity if you have the option of doing one or more on-site observations before starting your practicum. During an observation, you'll gain valuable information about the people who work there and the pace at which they work. Is it a friendly, service-oriented facility? How do the employees interact with their coworkers, patients, physicians, and visitors? Is the environment fast-paced or slow-paced? Which type of environment would be most comfortable for you? Some students prefer a fast-paced environment and they get restless when things move too slowly. Other students prefer a slower pace and feel rushed if things move too quickly.

Regardless of whether you're assigned to a site or have some choices, it's a good idea to do some research before you get there.

- Review the organization's website and printed materials. The more that you know about the site, the better prepared you will be and the more at ease you will feel on your first day.
- Ask your instructor for permission to contact the site ahead of time. Speak with the site supervisor and introduce yourself. Confirm your practicum start date, the hours that you'll be there, and the site's dress code. Discuss with your site supervisor before your start date if there are days when you'll need to leave early for class or a prior commitment.
- Travel to the site a few days before your practicum starts. Note the travel time. What time do you need to leave home in order to arrive at your site on time? How much traffic should you anticipate? What if the parking lot is full? What if your bus connection is running late? Imagine the worst-case scenario and have contingency plans.
- On your first assigned day, allow sufficient travel time to arrive at the site at least 15 minutes early so you'll feel more comfortable and less rushed. You don't want to arrive late or appear unprepared.

Remember, you never get a second chance to make a good first impression.

THINK ABOUT IT

OBSERVATIONS, PRACTICUMS, AND JOB OFFERS

Some practicum sites won't accept students unless they've done an observation there first. This pre-practicum observation gives students a chance to check out the site before starting their practicums. More important, it gives the site a chance to check out the students before accepting them into the facility. If students make a poor impression during the observation, there's a good chance they won't be invited back for a practicum experience.

An increasing number of employers are now hiring primarily from the pool of graduates who did their practicums at the site. In some cases, new employees start with higher pay if they did their practicum at the site. Think about it. If you did your practicum at the site that hired you, you save them time and money. You're already oriented and ready to work. You're familiar with the staff, physicians, and patients. You know how the department or work unit functions and you can operate the equipment, perform the procedures, and handle the paperwork. You can "hit the ground running" when compared with someone else who might need weeks or months of work experience to ramp up to the level from which you started. This is just one more reason to impress the staff at your practicum site and aim for a job there at graduation.

During Your Practicum

Keep a small notepad with you and take notes. Write down questions that you may want to ask later on. When you think of a question, it may not be the appropriate time to ask it. For example, if you have a question about the way a physician performed a certain patient procedure, it would be inappropriate to ask in front of the patient. Asking in front of the patient could make the patient feel uncomfortable as well as the physician. You may have questions that you want to hold until you meet with your program instructor again. During the course of a week, many things will happen and your notepad will really come in handy.

Keeping a Journal

Consider keeping a **journal** (a written record of your thoughts and experiences) during your practicum. Some educational programs require that you keep a journal and include certain types of information. Your program may be required to keep a copy of your journal in your student file. In such cases, it is best to record your personal thoughts and emotions in a separate document or notepad.

To protect patient confidentiality, you should not mention patient names in your journal. Take a few minutes at the end of each day to record what happened, how you reacted, how you felt about it, and whether you

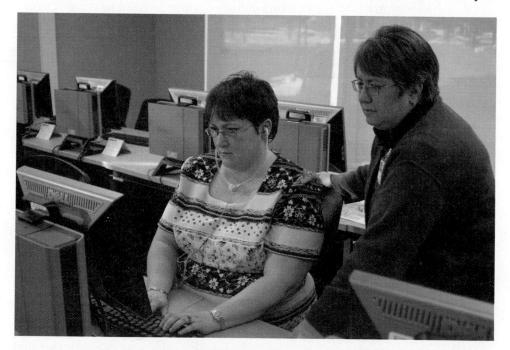

Figure 7-1 ■ Student functioning under preceptor supervision

could have handled it differently or better. Journaling can help you regroup your feelings, process your experiences, and reflect on what you've learned. Write about both the good and not-so-good things that you see and experience. Record both the things you do and do not want to do again in the future. Sometimes you may hear an employee being impolite to a patient. Write down what you heard to remind yourself how others may perceive the things that you say.

You'll likely see some things being done in a different way than how you were taught. By recording this, you'll remember to bring it up when you meet with your instructor and classmates later on. Expect to be nervous and busy at the same time. If you don't write things down, you may forget something important. If it's written in your journal, you'll have it as a reference whenever you need it. There are also some good pocket-sized reference books for different professions. Check with your instructor to find out if such a book might be helpful during your practicum.

Protocol

Your site will have policies and procedures outlining what you may and may not do as a student. These policies and procedures are called **protocol** and they will vary from site to site. Familiarize yourself with these at the beginning of your practicum and comply with them. Find out how the site handles cell phones and computer use. Some sites won't allow students or staff to use personal cell phones during work hours. In some situations, cell phones may interfere with technical equipment. Avoid making personal telephone calls and texting during your practicum hours. Keep in mind that the site's computers may be strictly limited to business use. It's always wise to ask before logging on to someone else's computer.

Depending on the profession and site, this may include getting permission from each patient before you are allowed to observe or participate in a procedure. Some patients are comfortable with having a student present during their procedure whereas others are not. As a practicum student, you must keep the rights of your patients in mind. You also have rights as a student including the right to observe and participate in procedures related to your educational experience. But the patient's rights always come first. If a female patient, for example, isn't comfortable with having a male student present during her procedure, the male student will need to comply with the patient's wishes. In most sites, there are a sufficient number of other patients who are comfortable with having students present to ensure that the students' educational goals can be met. Make sure you know how your practicum site protects the rights of its patients and comply with protocol.

Confidentiality

Maintaining confidentiality and adhering to HIPAA and the HITECH Act rules are top priorities. During your practicum you may have access to

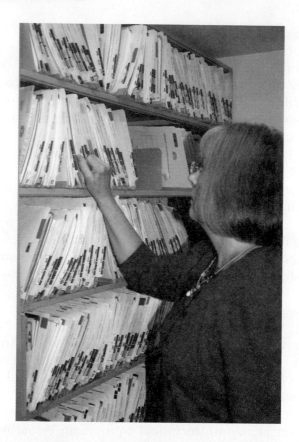

Figure 7-2 ■ Storing and retrieving confidential medical records

patient medical records and other private information. You may even know some of the patients. What you see, hear, or read at the site *must* stay at the site. Never read a patient's medical record unless instructed to do so. You will undoubtedly see and do things that you'll want to tell your family and friends about. It's natural to be excited and want to share your experiences. But you must remember to never use the patient's name or provide any other descriptive information that could reveal the patient's identity.

Here's an example of an acceptable comment:

You won't believe what I did today. We removed a mole from a patient's arm. I got to prepare the patient for minor surgery and assist the doctor with the procedure.

You described what you did without breaking confidentiality. Usually there will be times when you, your classmates, and instructor meet to discuss what you've seen and done during the week. Again, this is a time to protect the confidentiality of the site's patients.

In addition to medical records, you may also have access to other information such as patient financial records or the site's patient charges or financial transactions. This is information that must remain within the site and you should not talk about it with people outside the site. Private information is shared only on a need-to-know basis. This means the information is made available only to those people who need to know it to care for patients and conduct the site's business.

You may be rotating to different sites during your practicum and working in companies that compete with one another. Maintain the privacy of business-related information and use discretion when making comparisons among the different places you work. Remember what was said previously—you are a guest at the site and the supervisor has the right to terminate your practicum at any point should your performance pose a problem. Violation of confidentiality or the unauthorized sharing of sensitive information is a legitimate reason for immediate termination. If you are terminated from your practicum site, you might find it difficult to gain access to another site and your quest for recognition as a health care professional will suffer a major setback.

Samples

Many sites have what's called a **samples room**. This is a place (sometimes a closet) where they keep samples of drugs and medical supplies. You may be asked to go there and get samples of something for a patient. Just because the sales reps leave samples at the site at no charge, and the site gives samples to patients at no charge, you shouldn't assume that you can help yourself to anything that you want out of the samples room at no charge. Remember the practicum student mentioned previously who didn't get the job? One of the places she was discovered visiting frequently was the samples room. Needless to say, this behavior didn't support a positive reputation.

Office Politics

No discussion about proper behavior during during a practicum would be complete without talking about **office politics** (cliquelike relationships among groups of coworkers that involve scheming and plotting) and how to avoid them. If you've had more than one job, you've probably already discovered that all workplaces have office politics. Whether you're doing your practicum in a physician practice, long-term care facility, or hospital critical care unit, there will usually be coworkers who don't get along well with one another.

One employee may tell you something negative about another employee or complain about something that someone else has done. This happens frequently with students and it's easy to get caught in the middle. Stay neutral and don't get involved. Remember, you are not employed by the site and you probably don't have all of the facts. If you allow yourself to become involved in office politics, you may be labeled a troublemaker. The site supervisor may reconsider allowing you to remain there. You could be terminated from the site or lose your opportunity for a good employment reference or job offer at graduation. There's more to a practicum than just practicing your hands-on skills. Practicing your people skills and your professionalism skills are equally important in ensuring success.

One of the reasons sites agree to allow students to do practicums is that having a student present keeps the staff "on their toes." Students tend to be inquisitive and ask lots of questions. They watch how coworkers interact with one another and with patients, visitors, and physicians. The employees at the site are all aware of this. They must be able to explain things, answer questions, and set a good example. This helps keep the employees focused on the correct way to do things and cautious about their behavior.

More Than One Right Way

There is often more than one right way to do things and your way might not be the only right way. For example, when you clean a room, do you dust or vacuum first? It doesn't matter because both ways lead to the same result. If you observe a site employee doing something in a way that's different from the way you were taught, don't say, "That's wrong" or "You aren't doing that right" or "That's not the way we were taught." Instead, turn it into a learning opportunity. Ask the person to explain why and how he or she did it that way. You might learn a new technique that's easier and more efficient.

You will likely see different equipment in your practicum site compared with your classroom or laboratory at school. This is one of the benefits of doing a practicum. You get to experience different technology before starting your job. You should approach this situation by saying, "This machine is different from the one I was taught on. Would you please show me how this one works?" This sounds much better than saying, "I don't know how to work this machine. We weren't shown this in school." With the first example, you're indicating that you know the correct procedure but aren't familiar with the specific equipment. Medical equipment can be complicated to operate, mistakes can be expensive, and failure to use equipment properly can jeopardize patient care and patient safety, so make sure you know the correct way to use each piece of equipment.

Initiative

Once you've learned what is expected of you and you feel comfortable with the equipment and procedures, it's important to begin functioning with less direct supervision. If you are uncertain about something, by all means ask! But if you've been given a responsibility and it's your job to do it, then do it. If a patient has checked in and it's your job to escort patients to the exam room and take their vitals, then that's what you should do without waiting to be told. Don't make patients wait. If you hear the phone ring and you've been instructed how to answer it, you should answer it. The more you can do the better. The more you learn to do and the more cross-training you undergo, the more marketable you will become.

Keep one thing in mind. You are there to learn and to help, not to stand around and get in the way. Show initiative. One of the quickest ways to be labeled as unprofessional is to stand around doing nothing. Everyone from the receptionist to physicians will be watching your every move. Avoid spending too much time chatting with the staff. Be productive and help keep the site moving smoothly.

Language

Here's a story that actually happened in a large medical office. A medical assisting student reported to the office on the first day of her practicum. When she arrived, she couldn't remember the name of her contact person. As she was talking to the person seated at the receptionist desk, she became discouraged and used some **profane** (improper and contemptible) language. As it turned out, the "receptionist" was actually the office manager who was in charge of hiring for the practice. Needless to say, the student's practicum experience didn't get off to a good start and there was no job offer from the site at graduation.

Unprofessional language should never be used in your practicum site. That is not to say that you won't hear it yourself, because you will, but just because you hear the employees using profane language is no excuse to use it yourself. Put yourself in the patients' position. If you were sitting in the waiting room and heard the staff using profanity, how would you feel? What impact would it have on your opinion of the company? At each step of the way, put yourself in the patients' shoes. Even though you are there as a student, the patients will consider you part of the staff. Your behavior not only affects your own reputation but also that of the site. Using profanity or any other type of unprofessional language will undermine both reputations.

Teamwork

During your practicum, avoid becoming part of a clique. Depending on how long you're there, you may start to feel comfortable with the staff and feel as if you belong. Belonging is a good feeling but there's a difference between fitting in and being part of a clique. Fitting in simply means that you work well with the staff and you are viewed as cooperative. Your personality may blend well with the personalities of the employees, but being part of a clique can work against you. Cliques stick together and don't associate with the rest of the staff. They're exclusionary and they impede teamwork. Employees in cliques are typically less productive because they spend too much time socializing and gossiping.

CASE STUDY

Carla signed up for a free weight-loss program at work and joined a local fitness center using the discounted membership rates that her network provides for its employees. She's already lost 20 pounds and has more energy than she's had in years. After completing a health appraisal and getting good results on her blood tests, she qualified for a significant savings on the cost of her health insurance. Carla was so pleased that she treated herself to a new hair style and bought some nice business clothes. Now she's sure that she's making a more positive and professional impression on the people she meets and works with.

Carla has done so well since joining the practice that her manager decided to put her in charge of the three medical assisting students scheduled to do their practicums in the network. Her manager told Carla that she's a good role model for students. So once again, Carla has ventured into another new role with expanded job duties and responsibilities. She didn't get a pay raise but she's pleased that her manager has confidence in her abilities.

Carla has been thinking about what it takes to successfully supervise students. She's developed some leadership skills over the past year in her role with the Patient Experience team. But she's never taken a leadership course and she's wondering if she's really up to the task of supervising anyone, let alone students.

What could Carla do to gain more confidence in her new role? What would you do if you were in Carla's place?

Supporting teamwork should be one of your goals. When everyone works well together, the site can function smoothly. During your practicum, pay attention to which employees are good team players. Note the difference between team players and nonteam players. You'll notice that nonteam players have to work harder to get the work done whereas team players pitch in and help each other out. Strive to be a team player and avoid cliques. This could become a major factor in getting a positive employment reference or a job offer at the end of your practicum.

There are several other things to consider during your practicum. Protect yourself and others from communicable diseases by applying everything you've learned about infection control and standard precautions. Use protective devices and use them correctly. If you don't have enough respect to protect yourself, then you probably won't have enough respect to protect your patients and your site's employees. If you become ill during your practicum, stay home and don't report for duty. Avoid spreading your germs to the patients and staff.

Patient Preferences

During your practicum, you may come in contact with patients who are familiar with the staff and uncomfortable with anyone who is new, including

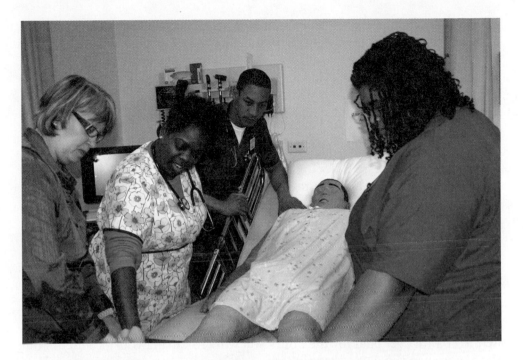

Figure 7-3 ■ Preceptor demonstration in a simulated environment

students. Don't take this personally because it's very common. Some patients will refuse to tell the student (or a new employee) anything. If a student tries to obtain the patient's history, for example, the patient may resist and ask for someone whom he or she is more familiar with. Patients can bond with members of their health care team and reject the involvement of people they don't know. If this happens to you, don't argue with the patient. Explain who you are and why you're there. If the patient still insists on interacting with someone he or she knows, simply excuse yourself and go get one of the staff.

Personal Issues

When you walk through the door to your practicum site, leave your personal problems outside. If you had a disagreement with your spouse or your child that morning, don't discuss it with the people working at your site. If you're upset, distracted, and not thinking clearly, you're more likely to make a mistake. Mistakes must be avoided whenever possible.

Never discuss your personal life or your own medical history with patients. You're there to focus on the patient's situation, not your own. The medical profession is a relatively small world. People who work for one company often know their counterparts at other companies. They participate in the same professional associations and attend the same continuing education conferences. When they get together, it's not uncommon for them to discuss personnel issues. If you're doing your practicum at a site where you don't want to work after graduation, just keep in mind that the people who work at your site may well know their counterparts at the site where you do want to work after graduation. Your performance and reputation as a student can easily spread from one place to the next without you ever knowing about it.

Ensuring Success on Your Practicum

Achieving success, especially during a lengthy practicum, isn't easy. Working without pay can become frustrating and tiresome, especially when you're a student with bills to pay and family obligations to meet. If your practicum occurs at the end of your educational program, you are probably counting the days until graduation and your first paycheck. When you look at employment ads, you'll notice that employers prefer to hire applicants who have work experience. Once you've finished your practicum, you'll have that experience. You'll know how the real world operates. You'll have firsthand knowledge and insights to share during your job interviews. You'll be more polished in your communication skills and you'll present yourself in a professional manner. You didn't get paid for the hours you worked during your practicum but the experience you gained is priceless.

Be sure to list your practicum experience on your résumé. Ask your site supervisor if you may use him or her as a reference. If you've had a positive experience, most supervisors will be happy to assist you in finding a good job. If you arrived on time, avoided unnecessary absences, and did your best to fulfill the goals of your practicum—and all without pay—then your site supervisor will assume that you will work just as hard or even harder when you are getting paid.

If you secure a job before graduation, and especially if you're hired by your practicum site, don't make the mistake of slacking off just because you've already landed a job. Too many students have made this mistake. Once they have a job, they start arriving a few minutes late, take longer breaks than they should, or fail to show as much initiative. This behavior indicates that they were making a good impression just to get a job. Keep this mind—the job that you already have becomes your reference for the next job you seek.

As mentioned previously, you'll probably receive a grade for your practicum. When you use your practicum site supervisor as a reference, he or she will be contacted by employers and asked a series of questions about you and your performance. The following criteria are the types of things that will be considered when assigning your grade and providing an employment reference:

1 *Were you dependable?*
Did you show up on time, ready to work? How many times were you absent? When absent, did you follow procedures for calling in? No matter how competent you are, if you aren't there, you aren't doing your

job. Employers would rather have a less-experienced employee with a good attendance record than an experienced employee with a poor attendance record.

2 *Was your appearance professional?*
Were you dressed appropriately and neat and clean? Did your appearance reflect a positive image to your patients and the site's staff? Avoid trendy clothing and appearance. You may think that hair streaked in purple is fashionable but it's not appropriate in a business setting. If you wear jewelry, make sure it's conducive to the work you're doing. Safety comes first when working with body fluids, equipment, and patients. Remember that some professions don't allow any jewelry to be worn for this reason.

3 *Did you display a friendly personality and provide good customer service?*
Did you get along well with patients, physicians, and the site's staff? Were you cooperative with the staff and a team player?

4 *How well did you work under stress?*
Did you maintain a calm demeanor and balance the priorities of your work appropriately? Did you adapt well to change?

5 *How well did you perform your duties with limited supervision?*
Did you demonstrate initiative or wait to be told what to do? Did you accept responsibility and perform your duties competently?

6 *Did you display a positive attitude and a desire to learn?*
Were you motivated? Did you ask good questions? Were you eager to learn new procedures and practice what you learned?

7 *Did you display a professional image?*
Did you apply everything that's been discussed in this book to make the very best impression you could possibly make?

If you can answer "yes" to all of these questions, you are well on your way to achieving a good grade, a positive employment reference, and possibly your first job offer.

After Your Practicum

On the last day of your practicum, thank everyone at your site. Let them know how much you appreciate the time they allowed you to be there and all of the encouragement and help they provided. Within a few days (no longer than a week) of leaving, send your practicum supervisor a handwritten thank-you note, which conveys appreciation and courtesy. Make sure you spell the person's name correctly and use good grammar and **penmanship** (handwriting). Believe it or not, thank-you notes can be the deciding factor in who gets a job offer and who doesn't.

If you apply everything you've learned so far in this book, you should have an exceptional practicum experience.

REALITY CHECK

Up to this point, if you haven't spent enough time gaining the knowledge and skills you need to be successful in your new occupation, your practicum experience will probably be disappointing. Your site supervisor is expecting you to be well prepared for your practicum. If you show up not knowing what you're supposed to know, your opportunity may be cut short. You may be sent back to your school to try to line up a different practicum site. If your skills are really weak, it's possible that no site may be willing to take you. Do you really want to get to this stage in your education only to be excluded from your practicum because you didn't take your studies seriously enough?

Health care companies that offer practicum experience don't exist to serve students; they exist to serve patients. Having students on-site provides some benefits for companies but many employers refuse to offer practicum experience for a variety of reasons. Supervising students, answering their questions, and showing them how to operate equipment takes time and results in an expense to the company. Students who perform poorly may damage equipment, waste supplies, and have a negative impact on the company's reputation and its patient satisfaction scores. When a company offers you a practicum experience, don't just take it for granted. The people who work at the site are taking a chance on you. If you perform poorly, you may be closing the door for future students who would like to do their practicum there. However, if you perform well, you may actually open the door for future students.

Key Points

- Research the site in advance and visit there before your first day.
- Keep a journal and use a notepad to jot down things you want to remember.
- Arrive on time and avoid unnecessary absences.
- Show initiative; ask questions and remember the answers.
- Dress appropriately and display a positive attitude.
- Show respect and put the site and its patients first.
- Remember that you're a student at the site, not an employee.
- Follow HIPAA and HITECH Act rules and protect confidentiality.
- Don't use profane language.
- Avoid discussing your personal life with the site's patients and staff.
- Don't participate in office politics or become part of a clique.
- Send a thank-you note shortly after your practicum ends.

Learning Activities

Using information from Chapter Seven:
- Answer the Chapter Review Questions.
- Respond to the What If? Scenarios.
- Complete Chapter Seven activities on the website.

Chapter Review Questions

Using information presented in Chapter Seven, answer each of the following questions:

1. Identify the purpose of a practicum.

2. List three benefits of a practicum experience.

3. Describe three ways to prepare for a practicum.

4. Discuss four examples of proper behavior while on a practicum.

5. Describe three ways to ensure success during a practicum.

6. Explain the importance of patient confidentiality during a practicum.

7. Discuss the value of keeping a journal during a practicum.

8. Explain the importance of putting the practicum site first.

9. Describe the connection between a practicum and employment after graduation.

10. Identify four general policies, procedures, and issues related to a successful practicum experience.

11. Define the term *protocol*.

What If? Scenarios

Think about what you would do in the following situations and record your answers.

1. While escorting a patient to the exam room, she asks you if her husband's tests results are back yet. You know that the results are back, but you don't have permission to give the results to anyone except the patient himself.

2. You notice the constant ringing of telephones in the office. You notice that the receptionist is talking on the telephone. But several times during the day, she's involved in personal calls. In the meantime, the ringing telephones are ignored.

3. One of your patients is a friend of your mother. She's at the doctor's office to find out if she's pregnant. After she leaves, her pregnancy test comes back as negative. You've been unable to reach her by telephone to give her the results. The next day you see her at the shopping mall with her family.

4. You realize that your neighbor is a patient at your practicum site. You see her medical record and are wondering why she always looks so tired all of the time. Her records are right there and no one is watching.

5. During your practicum, a patient mentions that he would prefer that no one other than his physician be in the room during his medical procedure. It's a procedure you've never seen before and you would like to observe. The patient will be under the influence of medication and probably won't remember what happened during the procedure.

6. You're short on money and need some antibiotics for your child. Her prescription has run out but there is a large supply of the same drug in your site's sample room. You notice that samples are given to patients free of charge.

7. While on your practicum, you notice that an employee has left work 15 minutes early every day for the past week. Two other employees who suspect this behavior but have not witnessed it themselves ask you to report it to the site supervisor.

8 Employment, Leadership, and Career Development

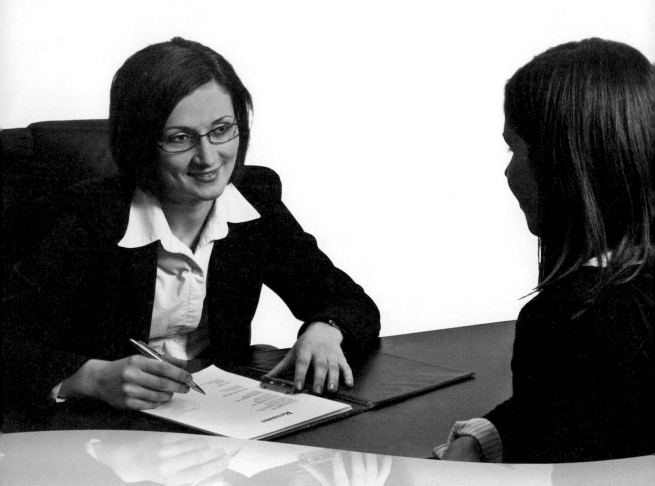

"My mother said to me, "If you become a soldier, you'll be a general; if you become a monk, you'll end up as the Pope." Instead, I became a painter and wound up as Picasso."

Pablo Picasso,
Artist, 1881–1973

CHAPTER OBJECTIVES

Having completed this chapter, you will be able to:

- List three sources of information on job openings.
- Describe four characteristics of a professional résumé.
- Name five things you should do when filling out a job application form.
- Explain why employers use pre-employment assessments.
- Describe five ways to present a professional image during a job interview.
- Discuss four characteristics of effective leaders.
- Identify two ways to develop leadership skills.
- List three benefits of joining a health care professional association.
- Describe five resources for professional development.
- Discuss the benefit of having a career plan.
- Define *role model* and *mentor* and explain the difference.

KEY TERMS

advocates

basic skills

behavioral questions

blogs

career plan

citations

clocking in and out

cover letter

credit report

criminal history background check

drug screen

dynamic

employers of choice

employment agencies

employment benefits

employment status

felony

full-time

hire-on bonus

human resources department

job application

job shadow

labor trends

legislative issues

long-term goals

mentors

misdemeanor

networking

occupational preferences

official transcripts

part-time

pathogen

perks

personnel department

portfolio

postsecondary

pre-employment assessments

professional development

reactionary

references

résumé

retirement benefits

role models

short-term goals

static

succession planning

supplemental

traditional questions

vested

vision

Job Seeking Skills

Finding a job that matches your qualifications and preferences is the next step in applying what you've learned in school. Job-seeking skills will help you identify **labor trends** (workforce supply and demand projections) and employment opportunities in the geographic area where you want to live and work. Once you have researched potential places to work, identified **employers of choice** (companies where people like to work) in your town, and developed your professional **résumé** (document summarizing job qualifications) and

cover letter (letter introducing a job applicant to a potential employer), you'll be ready to start contacting employers. This job-seeking process starts with learning the skills you need to find a job that's a good match for you.

Finding the Right Job for You

Looking for and finding the right job for you requires planning and job-seeking skills. In this chapter, you'll learn what steps to follow when you're ready to find a job. These skills will help you narrow down the type of job to look for and the most productive ways to spend your time finding it.

Where are the best employment opportunities that match your qualifications and **occupational preferences**—the types of work and work settings that you prefer? Your options will be somewhat governed by the discipline in which you are training. Depending on your chosen occupation, consider hospitals, outpatient facilities, home care agencies, community health clinics, rehabilitation facilities, physician practices, mental health centers, public health organizations, school systems, radiology imaging centers, laboratories, nursing homes, and surgery centers. You might be surprised at the variety of places that employ people with your education and skills.

There are a lot of things to think about when identifying your occupational preferences:

- Do you want to work close to where you live now or move to another location?
- Do you want to work in the same place throughout the year, work seasonal jobs in different parts of the country, or rotate among different companies as a temporary worker?
- Do you want to work **full-time** (working approximately 40 hours per week) or **part-time** (working approximately 20 hours a week) with **employment benefits** (employer-paid insurance and retirement savings) or do you want a **supplemental** job that provides flexibility in work schedules but no guaranteed work hours or employment benefits?
- Do you want a job where you can stay and grow with the company over time or just a place to launch your career?
- Do you want a small organization where you can become multiskilled and work in more than one area or a large organization where you can become a specialist?
- Do you want a job that pays well but may require compromising on some of your other preferences such as location, work schedule, or employment benefits?

Identifying your occupational preferences will help guide your job search:

- Geographic location (city, state, region, country)
- Type of employment setting (inpatient, outpatient, community-based, academic medical center)
- Size of the organization (small, large, statewide network, global company)

- **Employment status** (hired to work full-time, part-time, or supplemental)
- Work schedule and shift (days, evenings, nights, weekends, holidays, 10- or 12-hour shifts)
- Employment benefits (health, life, vision, and dental insurance; retirement and pension)
- Amount of compensation (pay) and paid time off for vacations, holidays, and sick leave.
- Opportunities for advanced training, tuition assistance, and job promotions
- Length of employment before eligibility for the company's retirement plan

Places to Find Employment Information

Once you've narrowed down the types of places you would like to work, investigate labor trends, job openings, salary ranges, employment benefits, and opportunities for career development. Labor trends forecast the supply and demand for different types of health care workers. Supply and demand changes over time and varies in different parts of the country.

When there is a shortage of nurses, for example:

- Demand increases.
- There are more nursing jobs to fill than there are nurses to fill them.
- Nurses have an easier time finding a job and may have several job offers from which to choose.
- Salaries and benefits increase to help recruit nurses.
- Employers offer a **hire-on bonus** (extra compensation for accepting a job offer) as part of nurse recruitment.

Conversely, when there is an oversupply of nurses:

- Demand decreases.
- There are more nurses looking for jobs than there are jobs to be filled.
- Nurses have a more difficult time finding a job and there is more competition.
- Salaries and benefits remain steady.
- Hire-on bonuses for nurse recruitment temporarily disappear.

Nursing shortages are predicted to worsen as experienced nurses retire and leave the workforce. Yet not too long ago, nursing students just graduating from school had difficulty finding jobs in many parts of the country. The situation is similar in other professions such as physical therapy, radiography, and respiratory therapy in which supply and demand cycles have shifted over recent years.

Locate specific websites and other references to help you monitor the labor trends for your profession. By tracking the supply and demand for people in your field, you'll know the best time to apply for a job and how difficult or easy it might be to find the kind of job you're looking for.

Identify which companies are considered the health care employers of choice in your area. Employers of choice do the following:

- Actively support the growth, development, and job advancement of employees.
- Provide scholarships, tuition assistance, on-site continuing education, and advanced training for employees.
- Offer flexible work schedules for employees enrolled in school.
- Host an Employee Assistance Program to help workers resolve personal issues and overcome barriers to job retention.
- Support a work environment that fosters continual improvement and lifelong learning.

If an employer has already helped you with a scholarship, part-time job, or other means of support while in school, show your loyalty. If the employer took a chance on you and invested in your education, then as a professional you have an obligation to repay that investment and work there for a sufficient period of time.

This is no time to take shortcuts in your homework. Make contacts with people who can help you investigate the best employment opportunities where you want to live and work. Landing your first professional job will launch your career and point it in the right direction. Making good decisions early in your career will increase your potential for a lifetime filled with satisfying and rewarding work.

Even if you're young, don't ignore the importance of **retirement benefits** (employer-funded pension contributions). You probably won't think about retiring for many years but your first job lays the foundation for your career and your life. If an employer is willing to invest in your retirement plan and perhaps even match the funds that you save yourself, you might be surprised how quickly those investments will grow over the years and provide a nice nest egg when you're ready to retire.

Here are some places to find information about job openings:

- *Internet.* Having access to the Internet is vital when seeking jobs in health care. Most hospitals and many health care organizations have websites and may post their job openings online. Check out professional association websites and search the key words *job search* or *job link.* You can find job postings, career fairs, workshops for job-seekers, and tips on writing a résumé and interviewing. You can also post your résumé online for potential employers to view.
- *Newspaper ads.* Get into the habit of reading the classified advertisements in local newspapers and online newspaper sites and track job opportunities from week to week. Look under "help wanted." There are different ways of listing jobs. Some papers list all health care positions under "medical." Others list them under a particular job title. Also become familiar with some of the abbreviations used by newspapers (see Box 8-1 ■).

Box 8-1 ■ Common Abbreviations

appl.	applicant	immed.	immediately
asst.	assistant	incl.	included
cert.	certified	lic.	licensed
exp.	experience	Suppl.	supplemental
FT	full-time	PT	part-time

- *Employment settings.* If you're looking for a position in a medical laboratory, apply directly to a laboratory. If you want to work in a hospital, go to the hospital's website or visit their **personnel department** or **human resources department** (people within a company who recruit, select, and employ job applicants). The Yellow Pages of your phone book offers an extensive list of possible employers.

- *Health care workers.* Speak with health care workers to get their opinions on the best places to work. They may have worked for numerous employers and can help you identify employers of choice in the area.

- *Networking.* **Networking** is interacting with a variety of people in different settings and can help strengthen your interpersonal skills, identify job opportunities, and uncover the best places to work. Join a professional association, become a volunteer, or participate in community activities to widen your scope of collegial relationships.

- *Friends and relatives.* You may know someone who works in health care who can suggest a place to apply or introduce you to a possible employer.

- *School counselors, placement coordinators, and librarians.* Schools often have resource people who can help you track down job openings. They're a good resource for information on current employment trends and how to find job openings where you want to work.

- *School bulletin boards.* If you have a career center or a bulletin board where jobs are listed, be sure to check it daily.

- *Occupational reference materials.* Reference guides available online and in libraries list the locations, sizes, and other helpful details for health care organizations around the country.

- *Employment agencies.* **Employment agencies**, some of whom specialize in health care, help connect job applicants with employers. Employers post their job openings with the agency and then job-seekers review the postings to see which might be a good fit. Public employment agencies are funded by tax dollars and don't charge a fee for their service. You can find public employment agencies online and in the White Pages

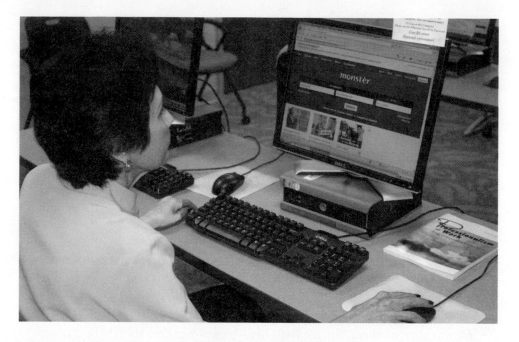

Figure 8-1 ■ Job hunting via the Internet

under "government agencies." Private employment agencies, however, do charge for their services. Some charge the employer whereas others charge the job-seeker. You can find information about private employment agencies online and in the Yellow Pages.

There are now hundreds of websites such as monster.com where you can find job openings, post your résumé, and apply for jobs online. Once you've set up your profile and posted your résumé, you can create alerts to e-mail you when new jobs have been posted. You can submit an application with the click of your mouse and keep track of the places where you've applied. Sites such as these can be especially helpful when looking for job opportunities beyond your region of the country.

Cover Letters

Now that you know where to look for a job, you need to know how to contact the employer and present yourself in a positive manner. If you have a lead on a possible job, you may choose to call for information. Give your name, identify the job you're interested in, and ask how to apply.

You may be asked to submit a cover letter as part of your application materials. Even if a cover letter isn't required, providing one is still a good idea. Many employers now use online, electronic systems to store and distribute each **job application** (an online or paper form used to apply for a job) submitted. Online job applications limit the amount of information and the kinds of information that you can submit. So your cover serves as your sales letter—a way to sell yourself to the employer in order to get an interview. Your cover letter should:

- Be neat and easy to read and reflect good grammar and correct spelling
- State what job you're applying for and how you heard about the job opening
- Give a brief overview of your education, experience, and qualifications
- Refer to your résumé or **portfolio** (collection of materials that demonstrate knowledge, skills, and abilities)
- Request a personal interview
- Give your address, phone number, and the best way and times to reach you

Résumés

In addition to your cover letter, potential employers need more details about you and your qualifications. This is accomplished by preparing a résumé. Even if a résumé isn't required, it's still a good idea to have one. If you lack significant **postsecondary** education (after high school) or work experience, you still have important information to share with potential employers.

Résumés provide:

- A snapshot of your background, education, and work experience
- Experience that relates to the job for which you are applying
- The qualifications you're presenting for consideration
- Visible evidence of your written communication skills

If you've never developed a résumé, you can find Microsoft Word templates on the Internet or books in your school library or local bookstore to give you some guidance and examples. You could also ask someone who writes or reviews résumés to assist you.

Your résumé should be:

- Typed, professional in appearance, and concise
- Available in multiple forms (print and electronic, such as a Word document)
- Easily faxed, scanned, sent as an e-mail attachment, or photocopied with good quality
- Printed on plain white paper with no borders or graphics
- Well organized and formatted, using bullets and underlining

Organize the information and make sure your grammar and spelling are correct. The most current information should appear at the beginning of each section. Emphasize your educational background, skills, and abilities that match the qualifications for the job. If you're a young person with little or no job experience and limited postsecondary education you can do the following:

- List some of your high school accomplishments and extracurricular activities such as academic awards, sports, orchestra or choir, science fair entries, perfect attendance awards, or participation in school organizations.
- Mention leadership roles, computer skills, seminars, or training sessions you've attended, certificates you've earned, and distinctions you've received.

Submitting supportive documents (copies of certificates, grade transcripts, or recommendation letters from an instructor or previous employer) is usually permissible but don't get carried away. Select one or two of the best items to submit with your résumé and save the others for your interview in case you get a chance to present them in person.

Applying for Jobs

There are several things to think about as you get ready to apply for jobs. It all starts with the job application form and how to submit it.

Job Applications

As with the résumé, the job application conveys a lot of information about you and is an important part of the employment process. If employers receive a surplus of applications for a particular job opening, the application is typically the first item they use to narrow down the applicant pool and screen applicants. Employers screen job applications to:

- Determine if your qualifications match those of the job
- Evaluate how well you read and follow instructions
- Assess your written communication skills, spelling, and grammar
- Decide whether or not to proceed with an interview

If you need to submit your application online, make sure you have the computer skills required to navigate the company's website and enter your information electronically. If necessary, ask someone who is familiar with the process to help you.

RECENT DEVELOPMENTS

ONLINE APPLICATIONS ON THE RISE

If you're required to submit your job application online, you must have an e-mail account. Log in on the job application website and set up your profile, username, and password. Employers can view this information, so make sure that your username and password are appropriate. Allow time to become familiar with how the computerized system works. Keep your electronic résumé handy and expect to cut and paste sections from your résumé to your application. With many online systems, you can save a draft of your application and go back later to revise and complete it. Pay attention to the knowledge, skills, abilities, and qualifications that are listed in the job posting and identify some of the key words. Use these key words in your application because computerized systems search for key words to find applicants who might be a good match. If you aren't familiar with completing online job applications, expect to encounter some challenges until you've learned how to navigate the process. This is especially true for people who have yet to develop some basic computer skills. If you fall into this category, take some computer classes as soon as possible. If the company where you want to work uses computers to manage job applications and the employment process, then they probably also rely on computerized systems for many other aspects of their business.

If the company uses a paper application form, fill it out yourself and don't ask someone to do it for you. Type the information or make sure your writing is legible and neat.

Regardless of whether you complete your job application online or on paper, you should do the following:

- Read the instructions and follow them.
- Use your best written communication skills and make sure all words are spelled correctly.
- List accurate dates for your education and work experience.
- List the job number if the employer uses a numbering system for job postings.
- Review the form to make sure you haven't left anything out.

If the application calls for a brief statement about why you're applying for the job, take some time to think about your answer before writing it. You might be surprised how much weight your answer carries in the selection process. Convince the reviewers that you're familiar with the job and their company. Let them know you believe that you're a good match for the qualifications they seek. If space permits, describe briefly how hiring you would benefit the company.

Your job application, cover letter, and résumé make that all-important first impression. Spend a sufficient amount of time making sure it's the impression you want conveyed. These three documents will likely determine whether you get invited in for an interview or not. Present your best attributes and don't undersell yourself. Stand on your own merits and avoid exaggerating your qualifications.

Be truthful—*never* falsify your information. Lying about your qualifications is dishonest, unethical, and unprofessional. If you misrepresent your qualifications and your lies are discovered, you will be disqualified as an applicant. If your dishonesty is discovered after you've started the job, you may be dismissed from the job.

THINK ABOUT IT

DISHONESTY ON JOB APPLICATIONS

Research shows that 70% of applicants overstate their qualifications on job applications. More than one-third lie about their experience and achievements and 12% fail to disclose criminal records. About a third of all job applicants admit to thinking about stealing from their employers. What happens when these applicants become employees? About half of all new hires don't work out, often the result of dishonest behavior before and during employment. The result can be devastating to the companies that hire them. About 30% of all business failures in the United States are caused by employee theft. Employee theft is growing by 15% a year and as much as 75% of internal theft is never detected. In addition to theft, work-related violent crimes affect about two million people every year.

If you've had a **misdemeanor** (a minor offense with a fine and/or short jail sentence as a penalty) or **felony** (a major offense with extensive jail time as a penalty) conviction, you must disclose it on your job application. Most employers conduct a **criminal history background check** (a review of legal records to search for misdemeanors and felonies) as part of the employment process. A prior conviction may or may not eliminate you from consideration depending on the job you're applying for, the type of offense, how long ago it occurred, and so forth. But if you fail to disclose the conviction and your employer discovers it later on, you could lose your job and do irreparable harm to your reputation.

Employers may run a **credit report** (a review of records to assess a person's financial status), visit social networking sites, and read **blogs** (similar to newspaper columns but published on the Internet instead of in print). Be very careful. Don't publish or share any personal information that you wouldn't want prospective employers to view or hear about.

Your job application form and résumé provide contact information that potential employers will use to set up an interview. Make sure that the recorded message on your telephone reflects the image you want to convey to potential employers. Think twice about religious, political, or musical overtones in your recorded message. Refrain from having children record the message or answer your telephone when you're expecting a call from a potential employer. An inappropriate, unprofessional, or confusing message may be all it takes to screen out your application.

References

Most employers require **references** (people who can provide information about job applicants). Choose your references carefully.

- One reference should be qualified to attest to your knowledge, competence, and potential for learning such as a teacher, program director, or practicum supervisor.
- A second reference should be qualified to comment on your character, work ethic, and reliability such as a supervisor or manager.

  Consider the following when lining up references:

- Select people who are familiar with your skills, the quality of your work, and your ability to learn quickly.
- Ensure the credibility of your references; never use a spouse or relatives as a reference.
- Contact people ahead of time and ask for permission to list them as references.
- When asked, provide written permission for references to disclose information about your performance.
- Identify the job you're applying for and when they might be contacted by the employer.

- Make sure you have accurate contact information for each reference, including their e-mail address.
- Choose references that have positive, insightful, and complimentary things to say about you.

If you know someone who works for the company to which you are applying, and if that person is familiar with you and the quality of your work, consider listing him or her as a reference. But avoid "name dropping, pulling strings, or using connections" to try to enhance your chances of a job offer. Such attempts could have a negative effect and backfire on you. Take the professional approach—stand on your own merits and get hired for the right reasons.

A frequent reason for terminating employees is poor attendance, so employers are especially interested in the attendance record of job applicants. Employers are typically impressed by job applicants who can demonstrate effective time management skills and the ability to balance school, work, and a personal life with good results. When an employer contacts your references for feedback about your performance and reliability, expect your attendance to be one of the topics brought up.

Another topic frequently raised during reference checks is your people skills. Employers need to know if you can form positive relationships with coworkers, perform well as a team player, display leadership skills when needed, treat people with respect and compassion, and display the personal traits required to deliver good customer service.

Choosing the right people as references and making sure they're well prepared to respond when contacted is critical. Employers often hold off checking references until they're close to making a job offer. If there's more than one finalist for a job, the applicant with the best references will probably get the offer. Even if you're the only finalist, just one less-than-satisfactory reference is all it takes to lose the job at the last minute.

CONSIDER THIS

BENEFITS OF ROLE MODELS AND MENTORS

Role models (people that a person aspires to be like) and **mentors** (wise, loyal advisers) can be helpful either as references or as advisers in helping you with résumé writing and navigating the employment process. Role models already have the education, work experience, and professional reputation that you aspire to achieve yourself. You can learn a lot from a role model because that person has already traveled down the road you are starting on. Mentors haven't necessarily achieved the same goals that you aspire to but they can provide the insight, advice, and encouragement that you need each step of the way. Consider who might make a good role model or mentor for you and ask if he or she would be willing to serve. You might be surprised how quickly someone will say, "yes!" Consider volunteering to serve as a role model or mentor for someone else. After all, everyone is on this road together.

Pre-Employment Assessments

Expect to take some written or computerized **pre-employment assessments** (tests and other instruments used to measure knowledge, skills, and personality traits) as part of the application and employment process. Employers need to know if your competencies and personal traits match the characteristics they're seeking. Some companies include an online assessment with their job applications. Other companies schedule half-day or full-day assessments to evaluate factors such as:

- **Basic skills** (fundamental aptitudes in reading, language, and math)
- Work ethic, character, and personal values
- Personality traits and customer service skills
- Job-specific skills (computer skills, applied math, and so forth)

Pre-employment assessments are difficult to prepare for because they measure the accumulation of the knowledge, skills, and personal characteristics that you've developed over time. When taking pre-employment assessments:

- Be well rested and ready to concentrate.
- Make sure you understand the instructions before taking the assessment.
- Try to relax and just do your best.
- Answer all questions in an honest and consistent manner.

Some employers will share assessment results with applicants whereas others won't. When an employer is willing to share the results, ask for feedback on how well you performed to learn about your strong and weak points. If your scores indicate some weaknesses, work on strengthening those skills as you apply for other jobs. If you don't get an interview the first time you apply, enhance your qualifications and reapply later. Some employers require a wait period of a few months before accepting another job application from the same person.

Verifying Qualifications

Most health care jobs today require a minimum of a high school diploma or a General Equivalency Diploma (GED). There are a still few jobs for people without a high school diploma or a GED but their opportunities for advancement will be very limited until they return to school and complete their high school education. Most health care jobs now require successful completion of a postsecondary training or college degree program as well as a professional license, certification, or registration.

Depending on the type of job you are applying for, you may need to submit supporting documentation such as an **official transcript** (grade report that is printed, sealed, and mailed directly to the recipient to prevent tampering by the applicant) from the schools you've attended; copies of diplomas, certificates of completion, or college degrees; and verification of active status of professional licenses, certifications, registrations, or other credentials required for the job.

Interviews

The personal interview is an extremely important part of job seeking. Taking ample time to prepare for an interview will payoff in the long run.

Preparing for an Interview

Once you've submitted your job application, résumé, references, and supportive documentation, completed your pre-employment assessments, and survived the screening process, it's time to prepare for your interview.

Making a good impression during an interview pulls together just about everything discussed in this book. The objective is to present yourself as a competent, motivated, caring professional who is well qualified and prepared for the job. Interviewers will be looking for information about your academic achievements, occupational experience, interpersonal skills, and personal qualities to help decide if you are a good fit for the company and the position. Don't just show up for an interview. Do your homework first.

RESEARCH THE COMPANY

Learn as much as you can about the job and the company ahead of time so you can talk intelligently about the opportunity for which you are applying. If you're applying for a job in an outpatient clinic, find out what kinds of patients are seen there, what services are provided on-site, what kinds of workers are employed there, what hours the clinic is open, and so forth. If it's obvious during the interview that you aren't familiar with the company, the interviewers will wonder if you're really serious about wanting the job or not. If you take time to research the company first, interviewers will be impressed with your interest and may give you some extra consideration in the selection process. To research the company you should do the following:

- Review the company's website, newspaper employment ads, and brochures.
- Read articles about the company online and in local newspapers and magazines.
- Find out if the company has won any recent awards or has been featured in special reports.
- Speak with people who are familiar with the company such as employees, patients, and vendors.
- Spend some time on-site before your interview to observe the environment.

Even if you've already answered a question on the application form about why you're applying for the job, expect to be asked this question again during the interview. Being familiar with the company and the job will help convince interviewers that you're a good match for the opening. Someone may ask, "What did you do to investigate this job and our company to make sure you this is a good match for you?" If you've done your homework, you'll have several examples to share with interviewers.

TYPES OF INTERVIEW QUESTIONS

Interviewers use traditional and behavioral questioning techniques:

Traditional questions ask how you *would* behave in certain situations.

Behavioral questions ask how you *did* behave in certain situations.

Many interviewers believe that past performance is the best predictor of future performance and that's why they use behavioral questions. Behavioral questions are more probing and call for more thought and specific answers. Here are some examples to illustrate the difference:

- *Traditional:* "What weakness would prevent you from being successful in this job?"

  Behavioral: "Describe a weakness you had in the past and explain what you did to overcome it."
- *Traditional:* "How would you handle stress in this job?"
  Behavioral: "Describe a previous stressful situation and how you handled it."
- *Traditional:* "What are your goals for the next 5 years?"

  Behavioral: "What were your goals when you started school and how successful have you been in accomplishing them?"

Once you've answered a behavioral question, expect more detailed follow-up questions:

- Why did you try that approach?
- What did you do or say that led to that outcome?
- How would you do things differently the next time?
- What did you learn from the experience?

Prepare for both traditional and behavioral questions because you won't know until you get there which approach the interviewers will use. It could be a combination of both types of questions.

Refresh your memory about challenges that you've faced, projects you've worked on, and goals you've achieved. Have some personal stories in mind in case you're asked for examples. Knowing as much as you can about the job description and the skills that your interviewer seeks will help you anticipate the types of questions that might be asked.

Practice at home or at school with someone firing questions at you in a mock interview setting. Be prepared to answer questions such as the following:

- Why are you interested in this job?
- Have you had a job that didn't turn out as expected? What did you do about it?
- What specifically have you done to investigate this job?
- How can you be sure this job is right for you?
- Have you ever been fired from a job? If so, why were you fired and how did you react?

- Have you experienced conflict with a former supervisor? If so, how did you resolve it?
- What do you think it would take to be successful in this job?
- What have you done to prepare for this job?
- Did you need to learn something new in your previous job? If so, how did you do that?
- What strengths would you bring to this job and this company?
- How did you support the reputation of the company you used to work for?
- What appeals to you about working for this company?
- Why should we select you over other applicants?
- Have you ever applied for a job and didn't get it? If so, what did you do?

The more questions you can anticipate in advance, the better prepared you will be. Expect some "what if?" questions such as the following:

- What would you do if you had to be late for work one morning?
- What would you do if you observed a coworker stealing from the company?
- What will you do if you're not selected for this job?

Interviewing is a two-way process. At some point during the session, the interviewer will probably ask, "What questions do you have for me?" You'll need to be well prepared for this because your response will carry some weight in the selection process. Here are some examples:

- Is this job full-time, part-time, or supplemental?
- What would my work schedule be?
- Does this job include employment benefits and if so, what are they (or where could I get more information about the benefits)?
- Once I'm on the job, what additional training or duties should I expect?
- Do you offer tuition assistance for employees who want to get more training or work on college degrees?
- How soon would I become **vested** (fully enrolled in and eligible for benefits) in the retirement plan?

When it comes to asking questions about how much the job pays, keep reading.

Participating in an Interview

The big day has finally arrived. Immediately before your interview:

- Review this chapter again to make sure the information is fresh on your mind.
- Get plenty of sleep and eat a good breakfast or lunch before your appointment.
- Make sure you know exactly where to go, how to get there, and where to park.

- Plan to arrive at least 15 minutes early.
- If you get delayed, call the contact person to let him or her know why you can't be there on time, apologize for any inconvenience, and ask if you need to reschedule.

Allow plenty of time for the interview itself. Other applicants may be scheduled for interviews during the same time period as you, so interviewers could be running late and you might be kept waiting.

It should go without saying but must be mentioned—don't bring children with you to your interview. Having children present is disruptive and an indication that you lack reliable childcare. If your childcare plans fall through, it's better to reschedule your interview than to arrive with your children.

Once you've arrived at the right time and place, it's important to make a positive and professional first impression. Your appearance will speak louder than words. Interviewers could be your age or younger but it's more likely they'll be older than you and perhaps about the same age as your parents. What type of clothing and personal image will they consider professional and appropriate for an interview? This is no time to think about styles and fashion trends or to wear something outrageous in order to be remembered or "stand out in the crowd." You definitely want to make a lasting impression but it should be based on your qualifications and friendly personality, not your unconventional appearance. Interviewers are going to "size you up" by assessing how well their patients, customers, business associates, and coworkers might react to you and your appearance if you were to get the job. So it's important to look your very best. The importance of wearing appropriate clothing cannot be stressed too much. Men should wear a suit or sport coat with a tie. Women should wear a business suit or professional-looking skirt, blouse, and jacket. Appropriate shoes and accessories are important. Avoid low necklines, ripped or baggy pants, or evening wear. Dress for success even if you have to borrow clothes.

Bring several copies of your résumé with you. Also bring your list of references with contact information that includes e-mail addresses. Make sure you have a notepad and pen. On the notepad, list some personal accomplishments and stories to recall in case you are asked. Jot down examples of how you've handled stress in the past and a situation in which you had to learn something new, in case you are asked. Have some questions ready to ask the interviewer when the opportunity arises. If you dropped out of school or have gaps in your employment history, be prepared to explain why.

Here are some documents to have ready:

- Your vocational portfolio, if you have one
- Thank-you notes from coworkers, patients, or physicians
- Awards or **citations** (honorable mention for receiving an outcome or result) that you've received
- Transcripts from courses, classes, and continuing education
- Copies of professional certificates and other evidence of your performance and professional growth

Bring copies of the most relevant items to your interview but don't overwhelm the interviewer with papers. Select just a few items that relate most closely to the job you're applying for and have them ready in case you need them.

Smile! Smiling is one of the easiest ways to make a good first impression. As soon as you are called into the room, thank the person for the interview. Don't sit down until shown a seat and until the person conducting the interview has been seated. Offer a firm handshake. Never hug the interviewer! Try to remember the names of the people to whom you are introduced. Apply your best interpersonal communication skills and personality traits. Remember the importance of customer service in health care. All health care employers seek job applicants with pleasant personalities who can relate well to other people. Practice your best people skills during the interview. It's okay to be nervous. In fact, interviewers might wonder what's wrong with you if you aren't nervous. But try to maintain your composure and self-confidence.

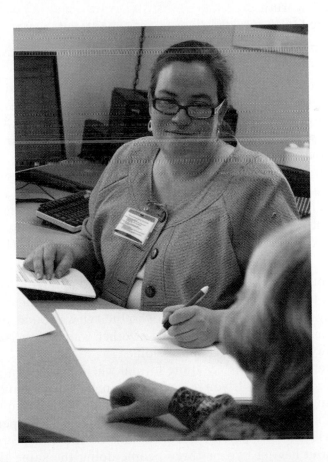

Figure 8-2 ■ **Manager conducting an employment interview**

During your interview:

- Describe the skills and abilities you would bring to the job.
- Convince interviewers that you would make a positive contribution to their organization and serve as an effective member of their team.
- Remember why you chose a career in health care; let your enthusiasm and commitment to helping people show.
- Be sincere; don't just make up answers that you think interviewers want to hear.
- Share some brief personal stories as examples of how you've overcome challenges and achieved your goals in the past.
- Be yourself; don't pretend to be someone you *think* would be more appealing to the interviewers.
- Trust the interviewers to recognize a good match when they see one; you want to be a good match for the job and you want the job to be a good match for you.
- Be honest; if you're asked why you left school or terminated employment, tell the truth.
- Be prepared to answer questions about your attendance, transportation, and back-up plans if things don't go as expected.

Here are some more things to think about:

- Sit up straight, don't chew gum or bite your fingernails, and try to relax.
- Pay attention to your body language and the nonverbal messages you are sending.
- Convey a positive attitude; don't express anger about a former teacher, job, or supervisor.
- Don't "carry baggage" from your past into what could become a new situation and fresh start.
- Display self-confidence and a genuine interest in what's being discussed.
- Don't ramble; stay on track and focus on the message you want to convey.
- Don't let your guard down; everything you say and do will be taken into account.

Even if you decide early in the interview that you aren't interested in the job, continue to put your best foot forward. A few years from now you may want to apply there again. The person who interviews you at one company may know the people who do the hiring at other companies. Never pass up an opportunity to make a good impression.

Some interview sessions are quite formal whereas others are more conversational and informal. If you're invited to lunch or dinner and it feels like a social setting, you are still being sized up as a potential employee. Don't be surprised if you're interviewed by more than one person, perhaps at the same time. Having one person fire questions at you can be intimidating enough without having two or three people doing the same thing during the same session. Sometimes employers have no choice but to have multiple people interview an applicant at the same time. Occasionally, it's done intentionally to see how well an applicant performs under pressure.

Answer questions thoughtfully. Concentrate on each question and think before you answer. Don't just blurt out the first thought that pops into your head but don't ponder too long either. Employers need to know if you can think and respond quickly. Let your interviewer know that you're always eager to learn new things. If you present yourself as someone who resists change, you'll likely lose points in the selection process.

Some interviewers ask intimidating, strange, or confusing questions just to see how applicants perform under stress. Don't let these kinds of questions shake your confidence. Interviewers are not supposed to raise the following topics during an interview:

- Age, race, ethnicity, religious, or political beliefs
- Marital status, number and age of children, and pregnancies
- Lifestyle preference (heterosexual, homosexual, bisexual, transsexual)

Unfortunately, some interviewers do ask inappropriate questions and then use the information to discriminate against job applicants during the selection process, so it's important to be prepared for these kinds of questions and have responses in mind. For example, an interviewer might ask a young female applicant, "When do you plan to start a family? How many children do you plan to have?" Or, "How old are your children and who takes care of them while you're at work?" With questions such as these, interviewers are concerned about the applicant's ability to manage parenthood and a full-time job at the same time. Which of the following responses would be most appropriate?

- You aren't supposed to ask questions like that so I'm not going to answer.
- I know that balancing my personal and professional lives will be a challenge but I've been working part-time and taking care of my elderly grandmother for the past 2 years while enrolled in school full-time so I know I have the skills and the support I need to manage a job and my family successfully.

It should be obvious which of these two responses would be best received by the person asking the questions.

Remember that interviewing is a two-way process. When the interviewer says, "What questions do you have for me?" consider asking:

- "What characteristics are you looking for in an ideal applicant?" (gather some important information and create an opportunity to describe how your qualifications match what the interviewer is seeking)
- "What is the potential for growth and advancement within your company?" (conveys that you are ambitious and seeking a company that you can grow with)

Jot down the responses along with any other information that you don't want to forget. Interviewers will notice that you're organized, pay attention to details, and record important information. Avoid asking for information that's already available in printed materials or on the company's website. Interviewers will wonder why you didn't do your homework.

Not everyone agrees on whether or not to ask questions about pay and benefits during the first interview. Although pay and benefits are important, it's best to focus on the primary responsibilities of the job and the qualifications being sought by the employer first. If you know there's going to be a second follow-up interview, wait for that appointment to ask about pay and benefits. Or let the interviewer take the lead in bringing up the discussion during your first interview.

Give some thought ahead of time to what your pay and benefit requirements would be in case you're asked those questions during your first interview. Saying, "I don't know" or "I haven't really thought about it" indicates you haven't done your homework. Before your interview, investigate customary pay ranges for the job you are seeking by using occupational reference materials, speaking with a placement adviser at school, or asking a human resources consultant or manager where you would be working. Keep in mind that pay rates are based on the geographic location of the health care facility.

How much pay do you need? It is okay to say, "The salary is negotiable" but have an acceptable range in mind in case you get pinned down or a job offer is extended. If you've done your homework, you've already identified what is most important in selecting the best offer. Instead of focusing on starting pay and benefits, new graduates should be more concerned about the job itself, support for continuing education, and opportunities to gain new skills and valuable work experience.

After the Interview

Regardless of whether you still want the job or not, you should follow up the interview with a letter thanking the employer for the opportunity to interview. This demonstrates courtesy and good manners and it also puts your name and communication skills in front of the decision makers one more time. Delivering a handwritten thank-you letter or sending a thank-you e-mail message within 24 hours after your interview will make a good impression because the majority of job applicants fail to follow up. Your thank-you correspondence also provides an opportunity to restate how excited you are about joining the company and to follow up on something discussed or forgotten during the interview. If you want the job:

- Contact the interviewer and ask if there is anything else you can do to verify your qualifications or answer any remaining questions.
- Try to wait patiently. It can take several weeks before employment decisions are finalized and offers are made.
- Avoid calling the interviewer to ask if a decision has been made yet. You don't want to become an annoyance or appear desperate. Most companies will notify all applicants when a position has been filled.

Expect some competition with other job applicants. When employers face shortages of qualified workers, it's easier to get a job and you may have several to choose from but when there's a surplus of qualified job applicants for the number of positions available, competition can be fierce. If you've mastered everything so far in this book, you should be in good shape to land the job you desire.

Considering Job Offers

Once you receive a job offer, it is decision-making time. You may even have the luxury of considering more than one job offer at the same time. To help ensure that this is the right job for you at this stage of your career, compare the offer with the list of important job factors that you identified earlier in this chapter. How well does the job match what you're looking for? Confer with your parents, teacher, adviser, or role model to help you analyze the situation and make the right decision. If this is your first health care job, you might not get everything you're hoping for. Identify your top priorities and consider making some compromises if the job might move you closer to what you're looking for in the future.

Once you've accepted a job offer, it will likely be conditional based on passing a pre-employment physical exam with a **drug screen** (lab test to detect illegal substances in a job applicant). Employers can ill afford to hire people with substance abuse problems. This is one example of when making a poor first impression usually won't result in a getting a second chance. As mentioned previously, some employers now also screen for nicotine and refuse to hire smokers.

If you don't get selected, you'll know you did your best and will have learned something of value in the process. If you believe you are well qualified, don't give up; employers value perseverance. Ask for feedback on how to enhance your qualifications, follow the advice, and reapply. It's not unusual for applicants to be turned down the first time and then hired later on. If you reapply and are turned down a second time, work with an adviser or mentor to revisit your goals and identify ways to increase your qualifications.

If you're seeking employment in a large or specialized facility or in a city or town where the competition for jobs is formidable, consider applying for a job in a smaller facility or in another city or town first and then making a move later on. Gaining work experience with a good reference someplace else may be the key to securing the job you really want. Graduating from school and landing your first job isn't the end of your journey, it's really just the beginning.

Becoming a Professional Leader

Once you've secured a good job and launched your health career, you'll need to start thinking about career advancement. It's never too early to plan ahead. Regardless of what profession you're in or where you work, developing some leadership skills is a great way to start working toward career advancement.

Leadership Skills

Similar to most other kinds of businesses, health care companies need people with effective leadership skills. Working in a leadership role can be stressful, but the rewards often outweigh the negatives. Successful leaders have the ability to articulate a **vision** (a mental image to imagine what the future could be), outline a plan of action, and direct individuals and groups toward common goals. Effective leadership is crucial in health care where the pace of change is rapid, the challenges are difficult, and the stakes are high. Health care is a complex life and death business. Its leaders must be capable, strong, dedicated, compassionate, empathetic, and sensitive to the needs of others. Leadership is providing the guidance, encouragement, and support that people need to achieve success.

The **perks** (benefits that come with status) associated with leadership jobs might look attractive, but there are good reasons why people in leadership positions often report stress and burnout. Effective leadership requires the following:

- Hard work and long hours to complete your own work while facilitating the work of other people; many leaders don't get paid overtime like hourly employees do
- Maintaining your technical and patient care skills while developing your leadership skills
- Communication skills to resolve conflicts among adults who really ought to behave better
- Managing stress while meeting impossible deadlines and attempting to do more with less and get better outcomes
- Being careful about everything you say and do
- Mastering new software, tracking emerging trends, and keeping up with industry developments

Unless you've been in a leadership position yourself, it's hard to imagine the stress involved in keeping so many different things in balance. It's easy to be critical of leaders who do things that you don't agree with or who don't respond as quickly as you would like. The next time you encounter leaders in your school or organization, think about what it must be like to walk in their shoes and consider giving them a break. Leaders are just like the rest of us, human beings trying to do their very best each and every day. No one is perfect and sometimes our leaders fall short.

Besides the drawbacks of leadership roles, there are lots of benefits to being a leader. Leaders typically:

- Receive higher pay than employees working at lower levels of the organization
- May be exempt from **clocking in and out** (using a time clock or electronic system to record hours worked) and have more flexibility in their work schedules
- Get more paid time off and work fewer weekends and holidays

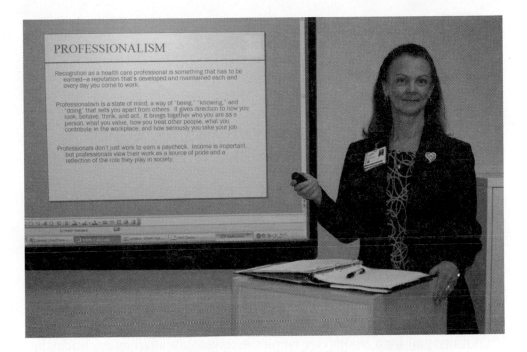

Figure 8-3 ■ Demonstrating leadership and presentation skills

- Have nice offices or cubicles, helpful assistants, and clerical support
- Get to attend workshops and go on company-paid business trips

However, many of the people who experience high levels of job satisfaction in leadership roles will tell you it's not the pay or benefits that make them look forward to coming to work each day. Leaders have the opportunity to:

- Articulate a vision, lay out a plan, and stimulate a collaborative effort
- Help the organization fulfill its mission and reach new heights
- Encourage people to learn, grow, and achieve their goals
- Make improvements to benefit employees, the company, and the patients

Creating and maintaining an environment that fosters excellence is an important aspect of leadership, especially in health care where quality outcomes are so important. Employees who work in an environment geared for excellence are more likely to take pride in their work, perform at high levels, and continually seek ways to improve patient care and customer service.

Leaders:

- Facilitate excellence among individuals and the group as a whole
- Provide the resources and tools employees need to do their work
- Act as **advocates** (people who speak or write in support of something) for individuals and the group within the organization
- Monitor the performance and outcomes of individuals and the group
- Adapt their leadership style to meet the needs of the group at any given time

In addition, effective leaders:

- Respect the rights, dignity, opinions, and abilities of others
- Display self-confidence and a willingness to take a stand
- Practice good listening skills and respect the opinions of those who disagree with them
- Value diversity and emphasize the benefits of individual differences
- Communicate effectively and state instructions and ideas clearly
- Are willing to work as hard as everyone else
- Complete tasks on time and according to expectations
- Display optimism and a can-do attitude
- Remain open-minded and willing to change and compromise
- Praise others and give credit where credit is due

Effective leaders don't expect subordinates to do something they aren't willing to do themselves. They openly support the company's mission, vision, and values and encourage other people to do the same. And they discuss matters privately when they disagree with a company policy or action.

Ways to Develop Leadership Skills

It's not unusual for a health care employee to get promoted into a leadership role before acquiring basic leadership skills. If this happens to you, you'll need to ramp up quickly. But if you have the luxury of time to prepare before moving into a leadership position, there are lots of ways to gain some leadership skills:

- Sign up for leadership classes, read some books, and review online resources.
- Work alongside an experienced and skilled leader and observe his or her behavior.
- Function as part of a team; observe other people's leadership skills as you develop your own.
- Volunteer to serve on committees at school, work, church, and so on.
- Participate in athletics, school clubs, and community organizations.
- Help organize special events and projects with family and friends.

All of these activities will provide valuable experience in working with other people and collaborating to achieve desired outcomes. Don't overlook the importance of being an effective follower. As mentioned previously, when you collaborate with other people you will fluctuate between leading and following based on the needs of the group at any particular time.

Becoming an experienced leader in your profession will take some time and patience. Here are a few places to start:

- Become well skilled and experienced in your health care discipline.
- Develop your critical thinking skills and learn to make thoughtful decisions.

- Strengthen your verbal and written communication skills and focus on conflict resolution.
- Learn about other cultures and develop respect and appreciation for people who are different from you.

If you have the opportunity, **job shadow** a health care leader to see what a typical day involves. Ask what types of skills are important and how he or she learned them. If you're interested in pursuing a leadership role, take some assessments to identify your strengths and weaknesses, enroll in classes to overcome skill gaps, line up a mentor who can give you some advice, and become active in a professional association.

Professional Associations

Becoming active in a professional association is one of the best ways to develop and practice leadership skills. Membership in a student organization or a health care professional association provides the opportunity to gain knowledge and practical experience in working with a wide variety of other people.

Health care has numerous professional associations that help workers remain current with emerging trends, new medical procedures, and advancements in technology. Most of these organizations are discipline specific (nursing, dental hygiene, medical assisting, etc.) and have local, state, and national chapters working together on common goals. Belonging to a health care professional association provides:

- Opportunities to develop leadership skills through elected offices and committee work
- Updates on new medical procedures and technological advances
- Information on salary ranges, employment trends, and job postings
- Updates on current **legislative issues** (topics involving local, state, and national lawmaking)
- Interaction with other health care professionals
- Pooled funding to support improvements in the occupation or profession
- Influence as a united group to encourage positive change

You can find professional associations by checking Internet sites, reading professional journals, attending continuing education sessions, asking fellow colleagues, and reading reference materials about the profession. Consider participating in professional Internet organizations such as LinkedIn to connect with other people who share common interests and goals.

Career Development

Life long learning is a critical component of professional growth and development because all health care professionals must continue to learn at every stage of their health career. Health care workers have many opportunities for

CASE STUDY

Carla had a fabulous experience supervising her three practicum students. Two of the students got off to a good start and did really well. The third student needed some extra help but he finally pulled through. All three of them were hired within six weeks of graduation. Carla's manager told her that she was really impressed with how Carla had related to the students, especially the young man who needed help overcoming the rough spots.

As a result of working with the students, Carla is even more excited about being back in school herself. She's been taking prerequisite courses toward a bachelor's degree but she's not sure what she wants to major in. Business management? With health care reform on the horizon, she'd like to learn more to help her network prepare for the new world in health care. Nursing school? Carla loves working with patients and has always dreamed of becoming a registered nurse. Education? Working with the students was challenging yet enjoyable. It took her back to her own days as a student and made her think seriously about becoming an instructor herself.

So many choices but which one is right for Carla at this stage of her career? Where is her career headed? What goals does she need to set for the next 5 to 8 years of her life? Should she go into management, stay in patient care and apply to nursing school, major in education, or follow some other career track?

Carla knows that her hard work has already paid off. That's why she now has so many career options from which to choose. She always gets the highest possible scores on her performance evaluations. She gets along well with everyone and has earned respect and admiration. She makes a positive first impression and maintains her reputation as a professional. She's committed to personal and professional growth and lifelong learning.

No matter what Carla decides to do next, she's pretty confident that she'll achieve her goals. She attributes much of her success thus far to a textbook she read in school called *Professionalism in Health Care: A Primer for Career Success*. She liked the book so much that she gave each of her students a copy when they started their practicum. She told them, "This is your roadmap to success. The information in this text will help guide your journey to recognition as a health care professional. Your patients will be counting on you. Nothing less is acceptable." Now Carla is ready to embark on yet another journey in her own career. She's not exactly sure where she's headed but she's thinking about starting to blog. Stay tuned . . .

professional development (education for people who have begun their careers and need to continue growing) through involvement in professional associations, employer- and college-based training programs and courses, and working with mentors and role models. Developing **short-term goals** (aims that will take a relatively short time to achieve) and **long-term goals** (aims that will take a relatively long time to achieve) as part of a well-constructed **career plan** (strategy for a person's professional growth and development) helps people identify next steps and stay on track. Health care professionals should always be on the lookout for new opportunities and anticipate revising their career plan periodically.

Reasons to Grow as a Professional

Why must health care professionals be life-long learners?

- *Ethical behavior demands it.* If you are to provide the best, most up-to-date service to your patients, you need to learn the latest developments in your field. Providing outdated, substandard care would be unethical and dangerous. In fact, many licensed professionals, such as doctors, nurses, and EMTs, must participate in a specific number of hours of continuing education each year to maintain their license.
- *Technology changes.* Medical technology changes rapidly. Diagnostic equipment that was unavailable a generation ago is part of routine medical care today. Computers and software programs are more important than ever before. Advancements in technology enable professionals to provide new services and better care to patients but only when professionals learn to use the technology safely and effectively.
- *Patient needs change.* The population you serve as a health care professional is **dynamic** (in motion, energetic and vigorous). As the number of elderly people increases, you'll need to learn more about geriatrics and the health care needs of seniors. If you work in direct patient care and a new disease or **pathogen** (micro-organism or virus that can cause disease) emerges, you'll need to learn as much as you can about this recent development and how to treat your patients while protecting yourself.
- *Responsibilities increase.* To advance in your career, you'll need more knowledge and additional skills to manage your new responsibilities. For example, you might need to learn how to read budget reports, interview job applicants, or increase productivity.
- *Job descriptions change.* Nothing is **static** (stationary and motionless) when it comes to job duties in health care.

Employers constantly reorganize departments, redesign work, and reassign staff. As the organization changes, so do job titles, job descriptions, and job duties. When jobs become obsolete, they are replaced by new jobs. Two jobs might be merged into one and employees undergo cross-training to work in both areas. To maintain your current job and to prepare for advancement, expect to always be involved in professional development activities.

Resources for Professional Development

Where can you get professional development? There are many resources available for the professional development of people working in health care:

- *Associations.* Many professional associations provide meetings, courses, workshops, journals, online modules, and other opportunities for professional development.

- *Employer training courses.* Many employers offer training courses to develop their employees. Employer programs include classes to improve customer service, communication skills, computer literacy, and competence in using new equipment and software. Employers may also offer tuition assistance for employees who wish to return to school and work on advanced degrees and professional certifications. In some cases a work commitment may be required to repay the investment the company has made in the employee's education.
- *Colleges and universities.* Many colleges and universities offer classes that can help you learn more about your profession. Lots of courses are now offered online for the convenience of working professionals.
- *Journals.* Professional journals help alert people to the latest developments in their fields. Journals also provide opportunities for health care professionals to write articles and become published authors.

Your Career Plan

A career plan is a strategy for your growth and development as a health care professional. Developing a plan requires forethought about the current status of your career, where you wish to be within a few years, what steps you need to take to achieve your goals, and what obstacles you might encounter along the way.

Some health care companies encourage or require their employees to have a career plan. The plan might be developed by the employee, with input

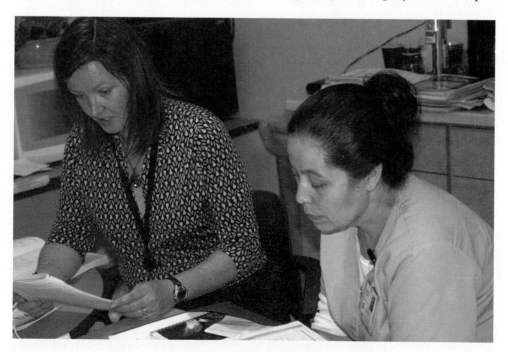

Figure 8-4 ■ Career planning with a mentor's assistance

from his or her supervisor to make sure the individual's goals align with the company's business goals. The plan outlines the knowledge and skills the employee expects to acquire during the coming year with specific learning and performance goals identified. When it's time for the employee's annual performance evaluation, his or her performance will be rated at least in part by how well he or she achieved the goals that were set.

It's still important to have a career plan even if your employer doesn't require one. You need to have a pretty good idea about where you are headed and how you're going to get there. Otherwise you'll be in a **reactionary** mode (responding to a stimulus or influence) instead of planning ahead. Many health occupations have career ladders for workers to climb, moving from entry-level jobs to higher-skilled jobs and potentially into more specialized jobs requiring additional education and credentials. In some occupations you can also move laterally instead of up the ladder, broadening your knowledge and skills. Identify the career ladders available in your occupation and think about what direction you might like to head in the future. It's your career, so take charge of it.

Whether you have your own career plan or a plan developed in conjunction with your supervisor, it's important to monitor your progress and make adjustments as needed. An increasing number of health care employers are actively engaged in **succession planning**. Succession planning is a proactive approach to identifying and preparing employees to fill positions when other workers retire. As the health care workforce ages and more employees begin to retire, employers must have a steady supply of well-qualified people ready to step in and take their place. Retirements create opportunities for advancement, so it's important that you plan ahead and be ready when these doors open for you. This is another reason why collaborative career planning with your supervisor is a good idea.

Setting Goals

Just as you set some goals when you first started your health career, you should continue to set more goals as your career develops. As mentioned previously, goals are well-defined stepping stones that help you progress from where you are now to where you want to be in the next phase of your career. Short-term goals are attained in a relatively brief period of time—up to about 2 years—whereas long-term goals take much longer. Long-term goals often involve meeting some short-term goals along the way.

One way to think about professional development is to view yourself as the leader of your career. Leaders articulate a vision, outline a plan of action, and direct individuals and groups toward common goals. As the leader of your career, you should envision your future, set realistic goals, and assemble a network of classmates, coworkers, teachers, mentors, family, and friends to help provide encouragement and support on your way to success.

When setting goals, you should avoid taking the easy way out. Most likely you have the ability to accomplish more in your career than you ever imagined. Your network of supporters can help you identify your strengths and develop strategies to fulfill your potential.

Changing Careers

As time passes and you revisit your career plan, you might find that you are growing in a different direction than you expected. For example, you might have discovered that you really enjoy training people in a new skill and decide to make teaching the focus of your career. Or perhaps you liked participating in a research project and decide to pursue research as a career track. Working in direct patient care for a prolonged period of time can be emotionally and physically exhausting for some people, so switching careers to focus on education or research might be the answer.

People change careers for lots of other reasons, too. Some people get tired and simply need a change. Jobs may become outdated and replaced with other kinds of duties. Switching careers might open new opportunities for advancement. Sometimes people discover health occupations they didn't know existed and decide to make a change. If you decide you would like to change careers, use the same process to investigate your new career that you used to find your first one.

Balancing Priorities and Career Advancement

As you set goals and proceed with your career plan, keep your priorities in mind and strike a good balance between your personal and professional life. Take things one step at a time and try to avoid overloading yourself. Enjoy your life and spend quality time with family and friends.

It's not unusual for health care workers to wonder if the time they're spending at work and on career advancement activities is negatively affecting their families. They may be setting a good example for their children through hard work, self-discipline, sacrifice, and perseverance. But balancing the goals of a dynamic career with the demands of a busy personal life is a challenge for many health care professionals.

Achieving your goals and reaping the benefits of a successful health career may require some adjustments. Don't be surprised if your goals change over time and don't become discouraged if attaining a goal takes longer than you had anticipated. Adjustments and delays are part of the process as you learn more about yourself, what you want out of your career, and what's going to work best for you and your family. The important thing is that you have a career plan with realistic goals and you're somewhere on the road to where you eventually want to be.

Expecting the Unexpected

Even if you are well on your way to achieving your goals, keep your eyes open for new opportunities when you least expect them. If options arise to train in a different discipline, move from an inpatient to outpatient setting, transfer to a new clinic or hospital within the network, or advance into a leadership role, seize the opportunity and let it work to your advantage. You never know what might be out there, just waiting for you around the next corner. It's all part of lifelong learning and the health career journey.

Expect to take some risks along the way. Risk taking *does not* mean being foolish or haphazard in making decisions but it *does* mean taking some cautious steps that force you to stretch a little bit. If you don't try, you'll never know what you can achieve.

If the going gets rough, don't give up. Talk with your network of supporters for encouragement. You'll probably hear that just about everyone else has gone through what you are going through. Most people think about giving up at one point or another in their careers. If your goals are worth achieving, they're worth fighting for. So hang in there.

For More Information

Post Your Résumé and Search for a Job
> www.monster.com
> 800-666-7837

Tips and Health Care Job Postings in Your Part of the Country
> www.employmentguide.com
> 877-876-4039

Labor Trends and Employment Projections
> Bureau of Labor Statistics, U.S. Department of Labor
> www.bls.gov/emp
> 202-691-5200

Resources and Tips for Job Applications, Cover Letters, and Résumés
> www.jobsearch.about.com

REALITY CHECK

When filling out job applications, developing a résumé, and participating in interviews, it's absolutely essential to be honest with everything that you say and do. There are plenty of examples of people who lied about their identity, education, work experience, credentials, or criminal history and got caught. Some of these people got caught before receiving a job offer. Others were already on the job before their dishonesty was discovered. In some cases, it might take an employer several months to realize that an employee had falsified information on his or her application.

If you lie about your identity or qualifications or fail to disclose personal information that would have disqualified you from employment, it really doesn't matter how long you're on the job before someone finds out. You can be fired at any time for fraud and dishonesty. In most health care companies, once you've been fired under conditions such as these, you won't get a second chance. You'll never be eligible for rehire.

It's small world. More than likely, your supervisor networks with leaders from other companies in your area. Once you've developed a reputation for dishonesty and fraud, word spreads. This is especially true in small towns or in geographic areas with a limited number of health care employers. All it takes is one dishonest act to make a negative and sometimes permanent effect on a person's future employment opportunities.

Key Points

- Identify your occupational preferences and labor trends where you want to work.
- Look for the best job opportunities that match your qualifications and interests.
- Include a cover letter with your résumé and job application.
- Make sure your résumé is accurate and conveys a professional image.
- Be honest and accurate in describing your qualifications.
- Disclose any misdemeanors or felonies on job applications.
- When applying online, allow time to learn how to navigate the computerized system.
- Expect a criminal history background check, physical exam, and drug screen as part of the employment process.
- Identify appropriate references and ask if they would be willing to serve.
- Line up one or more people to serve as your mentor or role model.
- Expect to take some pre-employment assessments as part of the job application process.
- Prepare for a job interview by having answers ready for the questions you expect to be asked.
- Present a professional image during your interview, including appearance and behavior.
- Develop some basic leadership skills as part of your professional development.
- Consider joining a professional association to support career advancement.
- Develop a career plan with short- and long-term goals and expect it to change over time.

Learning Activities

Using information from Chapter Eight:
- Answer the Chapter Review Questions.
- Respond to the What If? Scenarios.
- Complete Chapter Eight activities on the website.

Chapter Review Questions

Using information presented in Chapter Eight, answer each of the following questions:

1. List three sources of information on job openings.

2. Describe four characteristics of a professional résumé.

3. Name five things you should do when filling out a job application form.

4. Explain why employers use pre-employment assessments.

5. Describe five ways to present a professional image during a job interview.

6. Discuss four characteristics of effective leaders.

7. Identify two ways to develop leadership skills.

8. List three benefits of joining a health care professional association.

9. Describe five resources for professional development.

10. Discuss the benefit of having a career plan.

11. Define *role model* and *mentor* and explain the difference.

What If? Scenarios

Think about what you would do in the following situations and record your answers.

1. You've just graduated from school, moved to a new town, and need to find a good job. But you don't know anyone in town and you aren't familiar with area health care employers.

2. A new job just opened up but it requires some extra math skills. You're interested in applying but don't know if your math is strong enough to meet the qualifications.

3. You're planning to apply for a new job but your résumé is four years old. The new job is somewhat different from the one you have now but some of your skills might be transferable.

4. Your supervisor said she thinks you have leadership potential but you have no idea how to gain leadership skills.

5. You have a job interview at 8 a.m. Saturday morning. Your friends are having a party Friday night that starts at 9 p.m. and they want you to join them.

6. The job for which you would like to apply requires five years of previous work experience. You have three years of work experience in a large hospital that, to you, seems comparable to five years in a smaller hospital. A small change on your résumé would make you appear eligible to apply even though it wouldn't be totally accurate.

7. Last semester, your grade-point average dropped to a 2.0 (on a 4.0 scale) because you missed several classes while taking care of an injured family member. The company where you've applied for a job wants a copy of your transcript to verify your graduation. Because the company did not require an official transcript, it would be easy to change the 2.0 GPA to a 3.0. After all, your grades would have been better if not for missing several classes due to a family emergency.

8. After deciding to apply for a new job in an outpatient clinic, you find out your mother knows the clinic's human resource manager. Just a few months ago, your mother helped him refinance his home mortgage and your mother has offered to make a phone call to the human resources manager on your behalf.

9. The only interview appointment that's open is at 4 p.m. on Wednesday. You're scheduled to work at your current job up until 3:30 p.m. that day. Your supervisor has told you and your coworkers to wear old clothes that day because you'll be moving supplies and setting up a new inventory room.

10. You've applied for the same job twice and have yet to be selected.

PEARSON
myhealthprofessionskit™

Go to www.myhealthprofessionskit.com to access the Companion Website created for this textbook. Simply select "Basic Health Science" from the choice of disciplines. Find this book and log in using your username and password to access video scenarios, self-assessment quizzes, and more.

In Summary

Expect to encounter some bumps on the road to professional success. Some you'll navigate quite handily while others will require more maneuvering. At times you will soar and at other times you will stumble and perhaps even fall. After all, we're all just less-than-perfect human beings trying to do our very best.

Learn from your successes and your failures. Challenge yourself to always improve. Put your patients first and treat everyone you meet with respect and compassion. Face your future with courage and conviction, pause to appreciate the small things in life, and enjoy each and every step of your journey.

Best wishes for a stellar health career!

It is not the critic who counts, not the man who points out how the strong man stumbled, or where the doer of deeds could have done better. The credit belongs to the man who is actually in the arena, whose face is marred by dust and sweat and blood, who strives valiantly, who errs and comes short again and again, who knows the great enthusiasms, the great devotions, and spends himself in a worthy cause, who at best knows achievement and who at the worst if he fails at least fails while daring greatly so that his place shall never be with those cold and timid souls who know neither victory nor defeat.

Theodore Roosevelt,
26th U.S. President, 1858–1919

Glossary of Terms

accountability willing to accept responsibility and the consequences of one's actions (1)

accountable care organizations (ACOs) networks where hospitals and doctors work together and share accountability to manage all of the health care needs of a large group of Medicare patients for an extended period of time (1)

accreditation certified as having met set standards (Intro)

acute severe but over a short period of time (1)

adaptive skills the ability to adjust to change (6)

adverse effects unfavorable or harmful outcomes (1)

advocates people who speak or write in support of something (8)

alternative medicine using healing arts which are not part of traditional medical practice in the United States (1)

apps software applications for smartphones and computerized hand-held devices (5)

attitude a manner of acting, feeling, or thinking that shows one's disposition or opinion (Intro)

baby boomers people born in the United States between 1946 and 1964 (1)

basic skills fundamental aptitudes in reading, language, and math (8)

baseline data gathering information before a change begins to better understand the current situation (1)

behavioral questions ask how job applicants behaved in the past (8)

biased favoring one way over another, based in having had some experience (5)

blogs similar to newspaper columns but published on the Internet instead of in print (8)

body language nonverbal messages communicated by posture, hand gestures, facial expressions, etc. (4)

body mass index (BMI) measure of body fat based on height and weight for adult men and women (6)

breach a break, failure, or interruption (1)

capitation when a doctor, hospital, or clinic receives a fixed amount of money per person to provide health care services for that person (1)

career plan strategy for a person's professional growth and development (8)

caregivers health care workers who provide direct, hands-on patient care (Intro)

certification a credential from a state agency or a professional association awarding permission to use a special professional title; must meet pre-established competency standards (Intro)

character a person's moral behavior and qualities (3)

cheating deceiving by trickery (3)

chronic occurs frequently over a long period of time (1)

citations honorable mention for receiving an outcome or result (8)

civility politeness, consideration (4)

cliques small, exclusive circles of people (4)

clocking in and out using a time clock or electronic system to record hours worked (8)

colleagues fellow workers in the same profession (4)

comparative data information gathered from multiple sources that is analyzed to identify similarities and differences (5)

competence possessing necessary knowledge and skills (Intro)

complementary medicine combining alternative medical approaches with traditional medical practices (1)

compliance acting in accordance with laws and with a company's rules, policies, and procedures (2)

confidentiality maintaining the privacy of certain matters (1)

conflict of interest an inappropriate relationship between personal interests and official responsibilities (2)

conflict resolution overcoming disagreements between two or more people (4)

confrontation to face boldly, defiantly, or antagonistically (4)

conscience moral judgment that prohibits or opposes the violation of a previously recognized ethical principle (3)

consensus decision that all members agree to support (4)

constructive criticism viewing one's weaknesses in a way that leads to positive improvement (2)

consumers people who purchase or use a product or service (1)

contingency plans backup plans in case the original plans don't work (2)

continuity continuous, uninterrupted, and connected (1)

continuous quality improvement (CQI) the regular use of methods and tools to identify, prevent, and reduce the impact of process failures (1)

cooperation acting or working together for a common purpose (4)

corporate mission special duties, functions, or purposes of a company (2)

corporate values beliefs held in high esteem by a company (2)

corrective action steps taken to overcome a job performance problem (2)

courtesy polite behavior, gestures, and remarks (4)

cover letter letter introducing a job applicant to a potential employer (8)

credentials a letter or certificate given to a person to show that he/she has the right to exercise a certain authority (Intro)

credit report a review of records to assess a person's financial status (8)

criminal history background check a review of legal records to search for misdemeanors and felonies (8)

critical thinking using reasoning and evidence to make decisions about what to do or believe without being biased by emotions (2)

cultural competence the ability to interact effectively with people from different cultures (5)

culture groups of people who share the same values, norms, and behaviors (5)

data mining sifting through large amounts of data to find significant information (5)

defensive medicine medical practices aimed at avoiding lawsuits rather than benefitting the patient (1)

diagnostic deciding the nature of a disease or condition (Intro)

dignity the degree of worth, merit, honor (Intro)

diligent careful in one's work (2)

discipline a branch of knowledge or learning (nursing, medical assisting, surgical technology, etc.) (1)

discretion being careful about what one says and does (2)

discrimination unfair treatment of a person or group on the basis of prejudice (5)

dismissal involuntary termination from a job (2)

disparities lack of similarity or equality (5)

diverse different, varied (1)

diversity differences, dissimilarities, variations (4)

donut hole the gap in prescription drug insurance coverage that Medicare patients must pay themselves (1)

dress code standards for attire and appearance (6)

drug screen lab test to detect illegal substances in a job applicant (8)

dynamic in motion, energetic and vigorous (8)

emotional intelligence quotient (EQ) the ability to perceive, assess, and manage your own emotions and other people's emotions (1)

empathetic relating to another person's emotions and situation (5)

employers of choice companies where people like to work (8)

employment agencies companies that connect job applicants with employers (8)

employment benefits employer-paid insurance and retirement savings (8)

employment status hired to work full-time, part-time, or supplemental (8)

empowered to give authority, to enable or permit (1)

EMRs electronic medical records (1)

error something done incorrectly through ignorance or carelessness (1)

ethics standards of conduct and moral judgment (3)

etiquette acceptable standards of behavior in a polite society (4)

extenders people who assist other workers that are more highly educated and experienced (5)

extroverts people who focus on the outer world (5)

felony a major offense with extensive jail time as a penalty (8)

first responders the first people to appear and take action in emergency situations (5)

fraud intentional deceit through false information or misrepresentation (2)

front-line workers employees who have the most frequent contact with a company's customers (2)

full-time working approximately 40 hours per week (8)

gatekeepers people who monitor the actions of other people and who control access to something (1)

generalizations facts, patterns, and trends about groups of people that are backed up by statistics and research findings (5)

geriatric specializing in health care for elderly patients (1)

goals aims, objects, or ends that one strives to attain (2)

golden rule treat other people the way you want to be treated (4)

grammar system of word structures and arrangements (6)

gross domestic product (GDP) the total market value of all good and services produced in one year (1)

group norms expectations or guidelines for group behavior (4)

H-CAPS/HCAHPS Hospital Consumer Assessment of Healthcare Providers and Systems; survey to collect data about the patient's perception of his or her hospital experience (5)

hard skills the ability to perform the technical, hands-on duties of a job (1)

healing environment a physical space designed to reduce stress, ensure safety, and uplift the spirits of patients, visitors, and staff (5)

health care exchanges open marketplaces where buyers and sellers of health insurance come together to help consumers compare and shop for coverage (1)

health risk assessments questionnaires that identify which health issues you need to focus on based on your medical history and lifestyle (6)

hierarchy a group of people or units arranged by rank (Intro)

HIPAA Health Insurance Portability and Accountability Act of 1996; national standards to protect the privacy of a patient's personal health information (2)

hire-on bonus extra compensation for accepting a job offer (8)

HITECH Health Information Technology for Economic and Clinical Health Act of 2009; national standards to protect the confidentiality of electronically transmitted patient health information (2)

hostile workplace an uncomfortable or unsafe work environment (2)

human resources department current term for personnel department (8)

impaired a reduced ability to function properly (2)

inclusive a tendency to include everyone (4)

individual mandate a requirement that everyone must have health insurance coverage or pay a penalty (1)

infant mortality rate number of infants that die during the first year of life (1)

insubordination refusal to complete an assigned task (2)

integrity of sound moral principle (3)

intelligence quotient (IQ) the ability to learn, understand, and deal with new and trying situations (1)

intentional something done on purpose (2)

interdependence the need to rely on one another (2)

interpersonal relationships connections between or among people (4)

interpersonal skills the ability to interact with other people (1)

introverts people who focus on their inner world (5)

invasive   an assault or attack (5)

job application   an online or paper form used to apply for a job (8)

job shadow   observing workers to see what their jobs are like (8)

journal   a written record of a person's thoughts and experiences (7)

judgment   comparison of options to decide which is best (3)

labor trends   workforce supply and demand projections (8)

legibility   hand-writing that can be read and accurately interpreted by another person (1)

legislative issues   topics involving local, state, and national lawmaking (8)

license   a credential from a state agency awarding legal permission to practice; must meet pre-established qualifications (Intro)

life expectancy   the number of years of life remaining at any given age (1)

long-term goals   aims that will take a relatively long time to achieve (8)

loyalty   showing faith to people that one is under obligation to defend or support (3)

malpractice   negligence, failure to meet the standard of care or conduct prescribed by a profession (1)

managed care   a health care system where primary care doctors act as gatekeepers to manage each patient's care in a cost-effective manner (1)

manners   standards of behavior based on thoughtfulness and consideration of other people (4)

Medicaid   a government program that provides health care for low-income people and families and for people with certain disabilities (1)

medical homes   organizations that deliver primary care through a comprehensive team approach that ensures quality outcomes (1)

Medicare   a government program that provides health care primarily for people 65 and older (1)

mentors   wise, loyal advisers (8)

metrics   a set of measurements that quantify results (1)

misdemeanor   a minor offense with a fine and/or short jail sentence as a penalty (8)

mistake   to understand, interpret, or estimate incorrectly (1)

morals   capability of differentiating between right and wrong (3)

mortality rate   the ratio of deaths in an area to the population of that area, over a one-year period (5)

multiskilled   crosstrained to perform more than one function, often in more than one discipline (1)

networking   interacting with a variety of people in different settings (8)

non-compliant   refusing or failing to follow instructions (5)

norms   expectations or guidelines for behavior (5)

obese   weighing more than 20% over a person's ideal weight (1)

objective   what is real or actual; not affected by feelings (2)

observations   on-site learning experiences for students to view a "real-life" setting and take note of what occurs there (7)

occupational preferences   the types of work and work settings that an individual prefers (8)

office politics cliquelike relationships among groups of coworkers that involve scheming and plotting (7)

official transcript grade report that is printed, sealed, and mailed directly to the recipient to prevent tampering by the applicant (8)

optimists people who look at the bright side of things (2)

organizational chart illustration showing the components of a company and how they fit together (2)

outcome data information gathered after a change has occurred to examine the impact or results (1)

out-of-pocket expense costs that patients have to pay themselves (1)

outpatient a place to receive medical care without being admitted to a hospital; or a person who receives medical care someplace other than a hospital (Intro)

part-time working approximately 20 hours a week (8)

pathogen micro-organism or virus that can cause disease (8)

payer someone that covers the expense for goods received or services rendered (Intro)

peers people at the same rank (2)

penmanship handwriting (7)

people skills personality characteristics that enhance your ability to interact effectively with other people; also known as *soft skills* (1)

performance evaluation measurement of success in executing job duties (2)

perks benefits that come with status (8)

personal financial management the ability to make sound decisions about personal finances (6)

personal image the total impression created by a person (6)

personal management skills the ability to manage time, finances, stress, and change (6)

personal skills the ability to manage aspects of your life outside of work (6)

personal values things of great worth and importance (3)

personality distinctive individual qualities of a person, relating to patterns of behavior and attitudes (1)

personnel department people within a company who recruit, select, and employ job applicants (8)

perspective the manner in which a person views something (1)

pessimists people who look on the dark side of things (2)

polite courteous, having good manners (4)

political correctness eliminating language or practices that could offend social sensibilities such as race and gender (5)

portfolio collection of materials that demonstrate knowledge, skills, and abilities (8)

postsecondary after high school (8)

posture the position of the body or parts of the body (6)

practicum a "real-life" learning experience obtained through working on-site in a health care facility while enrolled as a student (also known as clinicals, externship, internship, hands-on experience, etc.) (Intro)

pre-employment assessments tests and other instruments used to measure knowledge, skills, and personality traits (8)

preexisting condition   when the patient has a medical condition prior to applying for health insurance (1)

prejudice   a judgment or opinion formed before the facts are known (5)

prenatal   occurring before birth (1)

preventive   actions taken to avoid a medical condition (1)

primary care   basic medical care that a patient receives upon first contact with the health care system, before being referred to specialists (1)

priorities   having precedence in time, order, and importance (3)

probationary period   a testing or trial period to meet requirements (2)

problem solving   using a systematic process to solve problems (2)

process   set of actions or steps that must be accomplished correctly and in the proper order (1)

procrastinate   to postpone or delay taking action (6)

profane   improper and contemptible (7)

professional associations   organizations composed of people from the same occupation (Intro)

professional development   education for people who have begun their careers and need to continue growing (8)

professionals   people with experience and skills who are engaged in a specific occupation for pay or as a means of livelihood (Intro)

protocol   policies and procedures (7)

providers   doctors, health care workers, and health care organizations that offer health care services (Intro)

punctual   arriving for work on time (2)

rational   based on reason, logical (2)

reactionary   responding to a stimulus or influence (8)

readmission   a quick return to the hospital after discharge (1)

reasoning   forming conclusions based on coherent and logical thinking (2)

references   people who can provide information about job applicants (8)

reimbursement   to pay back or compensate for money spent (2)

reliable   can be counted upon; trustworthy (2)

reputation   a person's character, values, and behavior as viewed by others (Intro)

respect   feeling or showing honor or esteem (Intro)

responsibility   a sense of duty binding someone to a course of action (2)

résumé   document summarizing job qualifications (8)

retirement benefits   employer-funded pension contributions (8)

role models   people that a person aspires to be like (8)

root cause   the factor that, when fixed, will solve a problem and prevent it from happening again (1)

samples room   a place where health care facilities keep samples of drugs and medical supplies (7)

scope of practice   boundaries that determine what a worker may and may not do as part of his or her job (Intro)

self-awareness   understanding where you are, what you're doing, and why you're doing it (2)

self-esteem   belief in oneself, self-respect (Intro)

self-worth importance and value in oneself (Intro)

sentinel event an unexpected occurrence involving death or serious physical or psychological injury, or the risk thereof (1)

sexual harassment unwelcome, sexually oriented advances or comments (2)

short-term goals aims that will take a relatively short time to achieve (8)

single-payer system when the government collects taxes for health care from all citizens and then uses the collected money to pay for the citizens' health care services (1)

Six Sigma a strategy that uses data and statistical analysis to measure and improve a company's operational performance (1)

smartphone a mobile telephone that has advanced computing and connectivity features (5)

social networking sites Internet places for people to publish and share personal information (2)

soft skills personality characteristics that enhance your ability to interact effectively with other people; also known as *people skills* (1)

specialists people devoted to a particular occupation or branch of study (1)

staffing level the number of people with certain qualifications who are assigned to work at a given time (1)

stagnant without motion; dull, sluggish (2)

stakeholders people with a keen interest in a project or organization; may be end-users of a product or service (1)

static stationary and motionless (8)

stereotypes beliefs that are mainly false about a group of people (5)

stress management the ability to deal with stress and overcome stressful situations (6)

subjective affected by a state of mind or feelings (2)

subordinates people at a lower rank (2)

succession planning a proactive approach to identifying and preparing employees to fill positions when other workers retire (8)

supplemental flexible work schedule with no guaranteed hours or benefits (8)

synergy people working together in a cooperative action (4)

systematic a methodical procedure or plan (2)

systems perspective stepping back to view an entire process to see how each component connects with the others (2)

telerobotics robots controlled from a distance using wireless connections; used in conducting remote surgery (5)

therapeutic treating or curing a disease or condition (Intro)

time management the ability to organize and allocate one's time to increase productivity (6)

traditional questions ask how job applicants would behave in the future (8)

traits characteristics or qualities related to one's personality (1)

transferable skills skills acquired in one job that are applicable in another job (1)

transparency open, clear, and capable of being seen (5)

trust to place confidence in the honesty, integrity, and reliability of another person (Intro)

trustworthiness ability to have confidence in the honesty, integrity, and reliability of another person (3)

unethical a violation of standards of conduct and moral judgment (2)

universal health care an organized health care system where everyone has health care insurance coverage (1)

up-code modifying the classification of a procedure to increase financial reimbursement (2)

vendors people who work for companies with which your company does business (Intro)

vested fully enrolled in, and eligible for, benefits (8)

vision a mental image to imagine what the future could be (8)

well groomed clean and neat (6)

whistle blower a person who exposes the illegal or unethical practices of another person or of a company (2)

work ethic attitudes and behaviors that support good work performance (1)

360-degree feedback feedback about an employee's job performance that is provided by peers, subordinates, team members, customers, and others who have worked with the employee who is undergoing evaluation (2)

Sample Job Description

Spruce Family Medicine Clinic
Greentree, IN

Job Title: Certified Medical Assistant
Job code: B254
Job family: Clinical
Pay range: MB7
Status: Non-exempt
Supervisory responsibility: No
Reports to: Office manager
Effective date: December 15, 2011

Summary

In addition to demonstrating core behaviors and standards of service expected of all employees, incumbent performs routine patient care and administrative procedures to assist physicians and nurses in examining and treating patients in a medical office setting.

Essential Duties

Essential duties include but are not limited to:

1. Greets patients, answers telephones, schedules appointments
2. Provides care to patients, prepares patients for examinations
3. Assists the physician during the examination
4. Explains treatment procedures to patients
5. Takes medical histories, records vital signs
6. Performs ECGs, removes sutures, changes dressings
7. Instructs patients about medications and special diets
8. Collects laboratory specimens, performs basic laboratory tests
9. Forwards prescriptions to a pharmacy
10. Updates and files patient medical records
11. Performs clerical functions and insurance billing
12. Maintains medical equipment and inventory of supplies
13. Maintains a clean, safe, orderly environment

Qualifications

Education: Graduation from accredited Medical Assistant program. Proof of high school diploma or GED. Certificate of Completion or Associate of Science Degree in Medical Assisting.

Experience: No experience required. One year relevant work experience preferred.

Certification: Certification by the American Association of Medical Assistants or the American Registry of Medical Assistants required.

Knowledge/Skills/Abilities

Incumbent will demonstrate the ability to:

- Perform and assist with diagnostic and therapeutic procedures
- Conduct medical office procedures and operate medical office equipment
- Communicate and document clinical and administrative information
- Apply knowledge of sterile technique, infection control, and safety precautions
- Apply age-specific competencies
- Establish and maintain effective working relationships with patients and staff
- Demonstrate good customer service and conflict resolution skills
- Establish priorities, organize tasks, and manage time efficiently
- Allocate and use resources cost-effectively
- Remain calm in stressful situations
- Display effective interpersonal and team skills
- Present a professional image as a representative of the practice

Computer skills:

- Demonstrate proficiency in Microsoft Word, Excel, Access, and Outlook
- Ability to perform clinic-specific computer applications and learn new applications and procedures

Additional qualifications may be required for any particular position. Employees may be expected to perform duties in addition to those presented in this description.

Sample Performance Evaluation

Employee name   ———————   Employee number   ———————

Job title/job code   ———————   Department/unit   ———————

Supervisor name   ———————   Supervisor title   ———————

Time period covered by evaluation: From ——————— to ———————

Date of supervisor meeting with employee (evaluation date) ———————

Rating Scale

Evaluate each performance factor using the following 1 to 4 scale:

4. Exceptional, consistently exceeds expectations
3. Effective, consistently meets expectations
2. Needs improvement, occasionally fails to meet expectations
1. Not effective, consistently fails to meet expectations

Part 1: Core Behaviors   **Rating**

1. Communication skills   ———
2. Teamwork/interpersonal skills   ———
3. Problem-solving skills   ———
4. Organizational/time management skills   ———
5. Respect for diversity   ———
6. Service excellence/customer service   ———
7. Support for quality improvement   ———
8. Support for cost-effective operations   ———
9. Support for corporate mission and values   ———

Comments:

Part 2: Personal Characteristics   Rating

1. Appearance _____
2. Attitude _____
3. Initiative _____
4. Adaptability, flexibility _____
5. Reliability, trustworthiness _____
6. Judgment _____
7. Ethics, integrity _____
8. Stress management _____
9. Accountability _____

Comments:

Part 3: Job-Specific Competencies   Rating

1. Greets patients, answers telephones, schedules appointments _____
2. Provides care to patients, prepares patients for examinations _____
3. Assists the physician during the examination _____
4. Explains treatment procedures to patients _____
5. Takes medical histories, records vital signs _____
6. Performs ECGs, removes sutures, changes dressings _____
7. Instructs patients about medications and special diets _____
8. Collects laboratory specimens, performs basic laboratory tests _____
9. Forwards prescriptions to a pharmacy _____
10. Updates and files patient medical records _____
11. Performs clerical functions and insurance billing _____
12. Maintains medical equipment and inventory of supplies _____
13. Maintains a clean, safe, orderly environment _____

Comments:

Part 4: Overall Performance

1. Attendance/punctuality   _____
2. Technical knowledge   _____
3. Quality of work   _____
4. Quantity of work, productivity   _____

Comments:

Part 5: Improvement Plans (if applicable)

Identify improvement plans for each performance factor rated 2 or below:

Part 6: Achievements and Recognition

List special achievements, awards, designations, or other types of recognition during this evaluation period:

Part 7: Goals and Professional Development Activities

List at least one measurable goal and a self-development activity for the upcoming evaluation period:

EMPLOYEE COMMENTS:

_____

SIGNATURES

Employee signature _____ Date _____
(Signature does not necessarily indicate agreement with evaluation ratings.)

Supervisor signature _____ Date _____

Approved by:

(Submit completed and signed original to Human Resources; copy given to the employee; copy maintained in the employee's departmental file.)

Sample Résumé

Jane Jones, A.S., CMA

123 Maple Street
Greentree, IN 47777
phone: 317-333-4444
e-mail: jjones@mail.net

Objective

Seeking full-time employment as a Certified Medical Assistant with clinical and administrative responsibilities.

Education

Greentree Community College, Greentree, IN
A.S. degree in Medical Assisting, April 3, 2011

Professional Certification

Certified Medical Assistant
American Association of Medical Assistants, April 20, 2011

Experience

Student Extern
Cherry Hill Pediatrics Center, Greentree, IN
December 1, 2010 to January 31, 2011
Poplar Grove Family Practice Center, Poplar Grove, IN
February 3 to March 30, 2011
Performed medical assisting clinical and administrative duties

Hospice Unit Volunteer
Greentree Baptist Hospital, Greentree, IN
June 1 to September 31, 2010
Answered telephones, delivered flowers, staffed the information desk

Nursing Assistant
Shady Dell Rehab Center, Elm City, IN
January 3 to May 30, 2010
Fed and bathed residents, assisted with recreation activities, filed
paperwork

Student Photographer
Greentree Gazette, Greentree Community College
March 15, 2011, to present
Produce digital photographs, attend editorial meetings, assist graphic
artists

Personal
Hobbies: horticulture, photography, antiques

Sample Résumé Cover Letter

Ms. Jane Jones
123 Maple Street
Greentree, IN 47777

May 20, 2011

Mr. John Johnson
Office Manager
Spruce Family Medicine Clinic
567 Spruce Street
Greentree, IN 47777

Dear Mr. Johnson:

I am writing in response to your ad for a Certified Medical Assistant which appeared in the *Greentree Reporter* on May 18. I am well qualified and eager to learn.

I have enclosed my résumé and am available for an interview at your convenience. Please contact me at 333-4444 or jjones@mail.net.

I'm looking forward to meeting you and learning more about employment opportunities with the Spruce Family Medicine Clinic.

Sincerely,

Jane Jones, A.S., CMA
333-4444
jjones@mail.net

Sample Job Application Form

It is our policy to comply with all applicable state and federal laws prohibiting discrimination in employment because of race, age, color, sex, religion, national origin, or other protected classification.

Instructions: Print clearly in black or blue ink. Answer all questions. Sign and date the form.

PERSONAL INFORMATION

First name _____

Middle name _____

Last name _____

SS number _____

Street address _____

City, state, zip code _____

Telephone number (_____) _____

E-mail address _____

Are you over 18 years old?   Yes _____ No _____

Are you a U.S. citizen or otherwise authorized to work in the United States on an unrestricted basis?

Yes _____ No _____

Have you ever been convicted of, or pleaded no contest to, a felony? (Conviction will not necessarily disqualify an applicant for employment.)

Yes _____ No _____

If yes, describe conditions: _____

POSITION and AVAILABILITY

Position applied for _____

Job number _____

Are there any hours, shifts, or days you cannot or will not work?
No _____ Yes: _____

Preferences:

Status   Part-time _____ Full-time _____ Supplemental _____

Shift   Day _____ Evening _____ Night _____ Weekends _____

Are you available to work overtime as required? Yes _____ No _____

What date are you available to start work? _____

EDUCATION

High school/GED Education

Have you earned a high school diploma or GED? Yes _____ No _____
Awarded by   _____
Date awarded   _____

Postsecondary Education (List all schools attended; use a separate sheet of paper if necessary)

School name   _____

School address   _____

Field of study   _____

Degree/diploma   _____

Graduation date _____

Other Postsecondary Education:

School name   _____

School address   _____

Field of study   _____

Degree/diploma   _____

Graduation date _____

Professional License/Certification/Registration

Title/date   _____

Awarded by   _____

Expiration date _____

Other Training and Skills:

Awards/Recognition:

_____

EMPLOYMENT HISTORY
(List all employment during the past 5 years; use a separate sheet of paper if necessary.)

Present or Last Position:

Employer Name: _____

Employer Address: _____

Supervisor's Name and Title: _____

Supervisor's Phone Number: _____

Supervisor's E-mail Address: _____

Your position:

Job title _____

Employment dates   From: _____ to: _____

Responsibilities   _____

Reason for leaving   _____

Previous Position:

Employer Name: _____

Employer Address: _____

Supervisor's Name and Title:

Supervisor's Phone Number _____

Supervisor's E-mail Address: _____

Your position:

Job title _____

Employment dates   From: _____ to: _____

Responsibilities _____

Reason for leaving _____

May We Contact Your Present Employer?

Yes _____ No _____

How did you learn of this opening? _____

Have you ever worked here before? No _____ Yes _____
If yes, dates of employment: From _____ to _____
Job title _____

References:

1. Name _____ Title _____

Address _____ Phone _____

E-mail _____

Relationship to you _____

2. Name _____ Title _____

Address _____ Phone _____

E-mail _____

Relationship to you _____

3. Name _____ Title _____

Address _____ Phone _____

E-mail _____

Relationship to you _____

I certify that information contained in this application is true and complete. I understand that false information may be grounds for not hiring me or for immediate termination of employment at any point in the future if I am hired.

I authorize the verification of any or all information listed above.

Printed name _____

Signature _____

Date signed _____

Sample Interview Follow-Up Letter

Ms. Jane Jones
123 Maple Street
Greentree, IN 47777

June 10, 2011

Mr. John Johnson
Office Manager
Spruce Family Medicine Clinic
567 Spruce Street
Greentree, IN 47777

Dear Mr. Johnson:

Thank you for the opportunity to interview with you and Dr. Seymour yesterday for a CMA position. Having met you and your colleagues and toured the facility, I am very excited about the prospect of joining the Spruce Family Medicine team.

I believe that my education, experience, and commitment to quality care and service excellence make me well qualified for the CMA position.

Thank you again for the interview and I look forward to hearing from you soon.

Sincerely,

John Johnson

Jane Jones, A.S., CMA
333-4444
jjones@mail.net

Sample Practicum Journal

Student's name: Jane Jones
Practicum dates: December 1, 2010, to January 31, 2011
Site: Cherry Hill Pediatrics Center, Greentree, Indiana

Week One

Day One

Arrived at my extern site for my first day at 7:45 AM. Was introduced to the physicians and staff and spent the day shadowing Dawn, the medical assistant to Dr. Moser. She showed me where everything was kept and I observed how she prepared the rooms for the doctor. This is a very busy office. I observed many different procedures and so far I am really impressed with how the back office and front office work together as a TEAM. Observed Dawn's technique at drawing blood. Her technique is a little different than our instructor showed us but she still used all the same equipment. Left the office at 5:00 PM.

Day Two

Again I arrived at 7:45 AM. Today I escorted all of Dr. Moser's patients to their rooms. I observed how Dawn assisted him with different procedures such as pap smears and skin tag removals. I also did my first blood draw on a patient. I was successful on my first attempt. Left the office at 5 PM.

Day Three

Arrived at office at 7:45 AM. Jumped right in and starting escorting patients to their rooms and preparing the rooms. Performed two EKGs today. Gave three injections and drew blood on several patients. Left the office at 5 PM.

Day Four

Arrived at office at 7:45 AM. Today I helped out in the medical records department as one of the women in the records department called in sick. Prepared and filed charts. Left the office at 5 PM.

Day Five

Wow, a whole week already! Arrived at office at 7:45 AM. Today we didn't have morning appointments until 10 AM. They invited me to sit in on their office meeting. Afterwards, I escorted patients to their rooms and assisted Dr. Moser. Worked in the lab in the afternoon, performed blood draws and UAs. Left the office at 5 PM.

Sample Practicum Thank You Letter

Ms. Jane Jones
123 Maple Street
Greentree, IN 4777

February 5, 2011

Dr. Martin Moser, Chief Medical Officer
Cherry Hill Pediatrics Center
456 Walnut Lane
Greentree, IN 47777

Dear Dr. Moser and Staff:

I would like to thank all of you for taking time out of your busy work schedules to allow me to complete the extern portion of my education in your office. I have learned so much by working with you. I know that having a student extern in the medical office can be a strain on everyone but the experience I have gained will make me a much better medical assistant.

Thank you for your time and patience with me during my externship. I am looking forward to applying what I've learned at the Cherry Hill Pediatrics Center.

Sincerely,

Jane Jones

Jane Jones, SMA
jjones@mail.net

Index

A

abbreviations, 177
accountability, 12, 33–34
accountable care organizations (ACOs), 12
acute, 3
accreditation, xv
adaptive skills, 142
adverse effects, 14
advocates, 195
aggressive communication, 86–87
alternative medicine, 10
American Recovery and Reinvestment Act of 2009 (ARRA), 39
appearance, 129–134, 129f, 131f, 165
application forms, 180–182, 227–230
apps, 107
ARRA (American Recovery and Reinvestment Act of 2009), 39
assertive communication, 87–90
assessments. *See also* performance evaluations
    H-CAPS/HCAHPS, 112–113
    health risk, 138, 138f
    personality, 105–106
    pre-employment, 184, 193
associations, professional, 197, 199
attendance, 33
attitude, xviii, 34–36, 75, 75f, 165

B

Baby Boomers
    characteristics, 106
    health care industry and, 6, 9–10, 9f
    workforce supply and demand and, 17–18
background check, 182
baseline data, 14
basic skills, 184
behavior
    diversity and culture and, 101–103
    illegal/inappropriate, 40–41
    practicum and, 156–165, 156f, 158f, 234
behavioral questions, 186–187
biased, 102
blogs, 136, 137, 182
BMI (body mass index), 138
body language, 84–85, 85f, 86f
body mass index (BMI), 138

body weight, 133
breach, 20
business etiquette, 80
business side of health care, 7–9

C

capitation, 12
career plan, 198
careers, 197–203. *See also* jobs
    advancement in, priorities and, 202
    changing, 202
    goal setting and, 201–202
    leadership skills and, 193
    life-long learning and, 197–199
    opportunities for, 3, 202–203
    planning for, 198, 200–201, 200f
    practicum and, 152–153
    professional development resources, 199–200
caregivers, as role models, xviii, 138
certification, xv, 38
change, managing, 142–143
character, 54–55, 55f
character traits, 55–57. *See also* personal traits
cheating, 58, 61–62
chronic, 3
citations, 188
civility, 78
clearance, gaining for practicum, 154
cliques, 76
clocking in and out, 194
clothing, 129f, 130–132, 131f
colleagues, 78
commitment, 28–32, 30f
communication, 84–94
    body language, 84–85, 85f, 86f
    electronic, 90–93
    listening and hearing and, 84
    with patients, 115, 117–119
    presentation skills, 93–94, 195f
    styles, conflict resolution and, 85–90
    teamwork and, 84
    written, 93–94
comparative data, 107
competence, xv, 36–37, 103–105
complementary medicine, 10
compliance, 37–40, 37f, 93
computers, 92–93, 107. *See also* Internet

confidentiality, 20
    electronic communication and, 91–93
    HIPAA and HITECH and, 39, 93, 157
    practicum and, 157–159, 158f
conflict of interest, 39
conflict resolution, 85–90
confrontation, 85–86
conscience, 59–60
consensus, 83–84
constructive criticism, 46
consumers, 7. *See also* customers
contingency plans, 33
continuity, 8
continuous quality improvement (CQI), 13–14
cooperation, 78
corporate mission/values, 41–42
corrective action, 33
courtesy, 78, 79
cover letters, 174, 178–179, 181, 226
coworker relations. *See* communication; interpersonal relationships
CQI (continuous quality improvement), 13–14
credentials, xv
credit report, 182
criminal history background check, 182
critical thinking, 31–32
criticism, constructive, 46
cultural competence, 103–105
culture, 101–103. *See also* diversity and culture
cultures, occupational, 108
customer service, 111–112, 112f, 165
customers
    coworkers as, 74–76, 75f
    doctors as, 119–120
    guests and vendors as, 120
    patients as, 111–112, 112f

D

data, 14, 107, 112–113
data mining, 107
dating coworkers, 136
defensive medicine, 12
dependability, 164–165
diagnostic, xvii
dignity, xvi

diligent, 36
discipline, 3
discretion, 43
discrimination, 110
dishonesty, 60–63, 62f, 181
dismissal, 33
disparities, 102
diverse, 3
diversity, 82
diversity and culture,
    101–110, 109f
  appearance and, 132
  behavior and, 101–103
  cultural competence, 103–105
  generational differences and,
    106–107
  occupational cultures, 108
  personality types and, 105–106
  respect and, 109–110
doctors, as customers, 119–120
donut hole, 11
dress codes, 129f, 130–132, 131f
drug screen, 193
dynamic, 199

E
education. *See* careers; practicum
electronic communication, 90–93
electronic medical records (EMRs),
    6, 18–20
e-mail, 90–93, 180
embezzlement, 61
emotional intelligence quotient
    (EQ), 4
empathetic, 115
employer, representing, 41–43, 42f
Employers of Choice, 173
employment. *See* careers; jobs;
    work ethic
employment agencies, 177–178
employment benefits, 174
employment status, 175
empowered, 16
EMRs (electronic medical records),
    6, 18–20
enthusiasm, 34–36
EQ (emotional intelligence
    quotient), 4
errors, 12
ethical dilemmas, 65–66
ethics. *See also* work ethic
  compliance and, 37–40, 37f, 93
  personal, 63–64, 65f
  professional development and, 199
  reputation and, 58
etiquette and manners, 78–81, 79f
evaluation. *See* assessments;
    performance evaluations
extenders, 108
extroverts, 105

F
Facebook, 136, 137
families of patients, 115–119

feedback. *See* performance
    evaluations
felony, 182
financial management skills,
    140–141
first responders, 107
fraud, 60, 62–63
fraudulent, 39
friendliness, 76–77, 165
front-line workers, 42
Fulghum, Robert, 78
full-time, 174

G
gatekeepers, 8
GDP (gross domestic product), 7
generalizations, 104
Generation X or Y, 106–107
generational differences, 106–107
geriatric, 18
goals, 44, 198, 201–202
Golden Personality Type
    Profiler, 105
golden rule, 76
grammar, 129, 134–135
green movement, 15
grooming, 129–130
gross domestic product (GDP), 7
group norms, 83
guests, as customers, 120

H
habits, 133–134
harassment, sexual, 39–40
hard skills, 4
H-CAPS/HCAHPS (Hospital
    Consumer Assessment of
    Healthcare Providers and
    Systems), 112–113
healing environments, 113
health, personal, 137–139, 138f
health care exchanges, 12
health care industry
  baby boomers and, 6, 9–10, 9f
  business aspect of, 7–9
  electronic medical records, 6,
    18–20
  occupational cultures, 108
  patient safety, 15–17, 17f
  reforming, 10–15
  role of professionals in, 20
  workforce supply and demand,
    17–18, 175
  working in, 2–7, 4f
health care reform, 10–15
Health Information Technology
    for Economic and Clinical
    Health (HITECH) Act, 39,
    93, 157
health insurance, 137
Health Insurance Portability and
    Accountability Act of 1996
    (HIPAA), 39, 93, 157
health risk assessments, 138, 138f

hearing, communication and, 84
hierarchy, xvi
HIPAA (Health Insurance
    Portability and Accountability
    Act of 1996), 39, 93, 157
hire-on-bonus, 175
HITECH (Health Information
    Technology for Economic
    and Clinical Health) Act, 39,
    93, 157
honesty, 60–63, 62f, 181
hostile workplace, 39
human resources department, 177

I
illegal behavior, 40–41
impaired, 30
inappropriate behavior, 40–41
inclusion/inclusive, 76–77
individual mandate, 11
infant mortality rate, 11
initiative, 160–161, 165
insubordination, 34
integrity, 55
intelligence quotient (IQ), 4
intentional, 31
interdepartmental teams, 82
interdependence, 29–30, 30f
interdisciplinary teams, 81
Internet
  health care resources, 107
  jobs via, 175, 176, 178, 178f, 180
  professional associations
    via, 197
  social networking sites, 31, 136,
    137, 182
interpersonal relationships, 74–81
  after hours, 135–136
  cooperation in, 78
  coworkers as customers in,
    74–76, 75f
  diversity and, 101–110, 109f
  etiquette and manners in,
    78–81, 79f
  inclusion and friendliness in,
    76–77
  language and grammar in,
    134–135
  loyalty in, 58, 77
  respect in, 109–110
  teamwork, 82–84
interpersonal skills, 4
interviews. *See* job interviews
intradepartmental teams, 81
intradisciplinary teams, 81
introverts, 105
invasive, 111
IQ (intelligence quotient), 4

J
job applications, 178–184
  application form, 180–182,
    227–230
  cover letters, 174, 178–179,
    181, 226

dishonesty on, 181
online submission, 180
pre-employment assessments, 184, 193
references, 164–165, 182–183
résumés, 164, 179–180, 181, 224–226
verifying qualifications, 184
job descriptions, 45, 199, 219–220
job interviews
follow-up, 192–193, 231
participating in, 187–192, 189f
preparing for, 185–187
job shadow, 197
jobs. *See also* careers
applying for, 178–184
considering offers of, 193
finding, 173–178, 178f
interviewing for, 185–193, 189f
opportunities for, 2–3
pre-practicum observations and, 155
skills required for, 3–4
journals, 156–157, 200, 232–233
judgment, 58–59

K
Keirsey Temperament Sorter (KTS-II), 105

L
labor trends, 173
language, 134–135, 161
laws, compliance with, 37–41, 37f, 93
leadership skills
careers and, 193
developing, 196–197
professional associations and, 197
qualities and benefits of, 194–196, 195f
teams and, 82
legal dilemmas, 65–66
legibility, 19
legislative issues, 197
less-invasive surgery, 111
licensing, 38
licenses, xv
life expectancy, 11
listening, communication and, 84
long-term goals, 198
loyalty, 58, 77
lying, 61

M
malpractice, 13
managed care, 12
management skills. *See* personal management skills
manners, 78–81, 79f
MBTI (Myers-Briggs Type Indicator), 105
Medicaid, 7
medical errors/mistakes, 12, 16

medical homes, 12
Medicare, 7, 60
mentors, 183
metrics, 14
misdemeanor, 182
mistakes, 16
moral dilemmas, 65–66
morals, 55
mortality rate, 11, 107
multiskilled, 3, 83
Myers-Briggs Type Indicator (MBTI), 105

N
National Patient Safety Goals, 16–17
networking, 31, 136, 137, 177
newspapers, jobs and, 176–177
non-compliant, 102
norms, 83, 101–105
notes, thank-you, 165, 192, 231, 234
note-taking, 156

O
obese, 10
objective criteria, 43
observations, pre-practicum, 154–155
occupational cultures, 108
occupational preferences, 174
office politics, 159–160
official transcripts, 184
online resources. *See* Internet
optimists, 34–35
organizational chart, 29
outcome data, 14
outpatient clinic, xiv
out-of-pocket expense, 11

P
part-time, 174
passive communication, 87
passive-aggressive communication, 87
pathogen, 199
patient care
cultural norms and, 101–105
focus of, 114–115
healing environments, 113
less-invasive surgery, 111
patient satisfaction data, 112–113
professional development and, 199
professionalism and, 29
Patient Protection and Affordable Care Act (PPACA), 11
patients
being there for, 114–115
communicating with, 115, 117–119
as customers, 111–112, 112f
family/visitors and, 115–119
pediatric, examination of, 118f
practicum and, 152–153, 157–159, 158f, 162–163

rights and responsibilities of, 110
safety of, 15–17, 17f
payer, xvii
PDSA strategy, 14
peers, 44
penmanship, 165
people skills, 3–4, 189
performance evaluations
elements and process, 43–47
during practicum, 153
sample evaluation, 221–223
perks, 194
personal etiquette, 79–80
personal financial management, 140–141
personal health/wellness, 137–139, 138f
personal image, 128–137
after hours, 135–136
appearance and grooming, 129–130
defined, 129
dress codes and, 129f, 130–132, 131f
habits and, 133–134
language and grammar and, 134–135
practicum and, 163–164, 165
social networking and, 137, 182
stereotyping and, 132–133
personal management skills, 139–143
financial management, 140–141
managing change, 142–143
stress management, 139, 141–142, 165
time management, 140
personal skills, 128
personal traits, 53–66
character and personal values, 54–55, 55f
character traits, 55–57
conscience, 59–60
ethics, 63–64, 65f
honesty, 60–63, 62f, 181
judgment, 58–59
reputation, 58
trust, 60
personal values, 54–55, 55f
personality, 4
personality types and assessments, 105–106
personnel department, 177
perspective, 20
pessimists, 34, 35
physical health, 141–142, 165, 193
physicians, as customers, 119–120
polite, 78
political correctness, 103
portfolio, 179
postsecondary, 179
posture, 129, 131

PPACA (Patient Protection and Affordable Care Act), 11
practicum, 150–171
    behavior during, 156–164, 156f, 158f
    behavior following, 165, 234
    benefits, 151–153, 160
    ensuring success of, 164–165
    journal, 156–157, 232–233
    preparing for, 154–155
    purpose, 151
practicum, xvii
pre-employment assessments, 184, 193
preexisting condition, 11
prejudice, 104
prenatal, 8
presentation skills, 93–94, 195f
preventive, 8
primary care, 8
priorities, 58, 202
probationary period, 43
problem solving, 32
process, 13
procrastinate, 140
profane language, 161
professional associations, xv, 197, 199
professional development, 198, 199–200
professional etiquette, 80
professionals, xiv
project teams, 82–83
providers, xiv
protocol, practicum, 157
public speaking, 93–94
punctual/punctuality, 33

Q
qualifications, verifying, 184
quality improvement, 13–15
quality of work, 36–37
questions, job interview, 186–187, 191–192

R
rational, 31
reactionary, 201
readmissions, 14
reasoning, 31
references, 164–165, 182–183
reimbursement, 39
relationships. *See* interpersonal relationships
reliability, 33–34
reporting illegal behavior, 41
representing your employer, 41–43, 42f
reputation, xvi, 54, 58, 137
research, 155, 185
respect, xvi, 109–110
responsibility, 34, 165, 199

résumés, 173, 179–180, 181
    practicum experience and, 164
    sample materials, 224–226
retirement benefits, 176
right thing to do, 64
rights and responsibilities, patient, 110
robots, 111
role models, 138–139, 183
Roosevelt, Theodore, 209
root cause, 15

S
samples room, 159
satisfaction data, patient, 112–113
scope of practice, xv, 37–38, 37f
security, computer, 92–93
self-awareness, 30–31
self-esteem, xvi
self-awareness, xvi
sentinel event, 16
sexual harassment, 39–40
short-term goals, 198
Silent Generation, 106
single-payer system, 12
site orientation, practicums and, 153
Six Sigma, 15
skills
    adaptive, 142
    basic, 184
    evaluating. *See* performance evaluations
    leadership, 193–197, 195f
    personal, 128
    personal management, 139–143
    presentation, 93–94, 195f
    soft *vs.* hard, 4
    transferable, 3
smartphones, 107
social media, 92
social networking sites, 31, 136, 137, 182
soft skills, 4
specialists, 8
staffing levels, 14
stagnant, 36
stakeholders, 7
static, 199
stealing, 61
stereotypes, 104, 132–133
stress management, 139, 141–142, 165
students, practicum and, 152
subjective criteria, 43
subordinates, 36
succession planning, 201
supercomputers, 107
supplemental, 174
surgery, less-invasive, 111
synergy, 78
systematic, 31
systems perspective, 29, 30

T
teams and teamwork
    consensus and, 83–84
    group norms and, 83
    occupational cultures and, 108
    practicum and, 161–162
    types of teams, 81–83
telerobotics, 111
thank-you notes, 165, 192, 231, 234
theft, 61, 62f
therapeutic, xvii
360-degree feedback, 44
time management, 140
traditional questions, 186–187
training courses, 200
traits, 5. *See also* personal traits
transcript, official, 184
transferable skills, 3
transparency, 107
trust/trustworthiness, xviii, 55, 55f, 60
Twitter, 136

U
unethical, 39
universal health care, 12
up-code, 40

V
values
    corporate, 41–42
    cultural considerations and, 101–103
    personal, 54–55, 55f
vendors, as customers, xvi, 120
verifying qualifications, 184
vested, 187
vision, 194
visitors, 115–119

W
Web sites. *See* Internet
weight, stereotypes and, 133
well groomed, 129
wellness, personal, 137–139, 138f
whistle blower, 41
work ethic, 5, 32–41
    attendance and punctuality, 33
    attitude and enthusiasm, 34–36
    commitment, 28–32, 30f
    competence and work quality, 36–37
    compliance, 37–40, 37f
    inappropriate behavior, 40–41
    reliability and accountability, 33–34
work teams, 82
workforce supply and demand, 17–18, 175
written communication, 93–94